Training Your Own Psychiatric Service Dog 2021:

Step-By-Step Guide to an Obedient Psychiatric Service Dog

written consent and can in no way be considered an endorsement

from the trademark holder.

Table of Contents

INTRODUCTION

Congratulations on purchasing *Training Your Psychiatric Service Dog 2021*. You are taking that first step to live a life with more freedom and mobility. A Psychiatric Service Dog allows you the ability to be more interactive within the world. It gives you the freedom to move about with the assistance that you need to have a fulfilling life.

They say that a dog is man's best friend, and I honestly believe that with the proper training, a dog can save a person's life. The dogs that are used as Psychiatric Service dogs are trained to be your best friend and your medical medium. They are trained to know what is going on in your life before you ever know what is going on. They are trained to be highly skilled at maintaining your health.

This book is designed to give you the tools that are needed for you to train your dog to be as skilled as any other Psychiatric Service dog. Even though I broke each training session into a specific diagnoses-based need, they can all be used to provide you with freedoms that you never thought were possible. Do not let your diagnosis get in the way of starting a new chapter in your life. Disability does not have to be the end of your life. It can be the beginning of a beautiful friendship between you and your Psychiatric Service animal.

The following chapters will discuss all the necessary steps that must be taken in training your own Psychiatric Service Dog. There are many skills and techniques in training a dog, and each one of these can provide you with more freedom and flexibility in your life. Psychiatric Service Dogs provide you the comfort of knowing that you can experience life and all its adventures without concerning yourself with those annoying disabilities that have been limiting you. Many people have found that with a Psychiatric Service Dog, they are able to spend more time out in the world enjoying concerts, restaurants, driving, and many other activities.

This is the book that will give you that freedom and peace of mind. Start training your Psychiatric Service Dog and begin enjoying life again in as little as 6 weeks.

There are plenty of books on this subject on the market, so thanks again for choosing this one! Every effort was made to ensure it is full of as much useful information as possible. Please enjoy!

CHAPTER 1: WHAT IS A PSYCHIATRIC SERVICE DOG?

Psychiatric Service Dogs are not pets, but a medical necessity for those who are suffering from severe Psychiatric Disorders. A Psychiatric Service Dog is a dog that is specially trained to provide a service for someone who suffers from a Psychiatric Disorder.

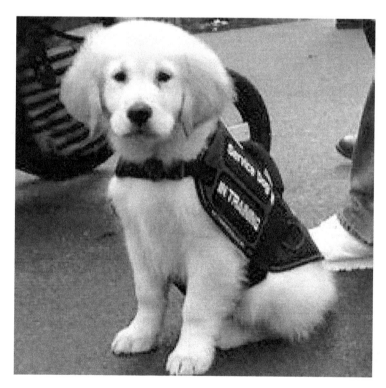

If you have a Psychiatric disorder, then you are well aware of what one is. If you do not have a Psychiatric disorder, then a little bit of information should help you understand if you have one. A psychiatric disorder is a disorder that is related to mental health. This can include anything from Anxiety, PTSD, Autism, Depression, Schizophrenia, and much more. If you have a disorder that limits your ability to live a fulfilling life, then you may need a Psychiatric Service Dog.

A Psychiatric Service Dog helps those with disabilities survive in a world that is unfriendly to them. It provides them with the ability to have life experiences that they would otherwise not have been able to due to their disabilities. They are able to have adventures and live a life without concern for whether or not they are going to have an episode.

Psychiatric Service Dogs are trained for many different services to assist the disabled in their daily activities as well as handling their episodes from their disabilities. These can be anything from alerting the owner to medication times, finding a lost item, checking the environment for triggers, recognizing an anxiety attack coming on, blocking the owner from being approached by others, calming them when in an episode, and many more services.

In this book, I will talk about what tasks are available for you to train your Psychiatric Service Dog to do, which types of dogs are best to train, the best age to start training a dog, different equipment that will help you with your Psychiatric Service Dog, the government rules and regulations for Psychiatric Service Dogs, what your Psychiatric Service Dog needs to know to qualify as a Psychiatric service dog, and a step-by-step guide on how to train for specific conditions.

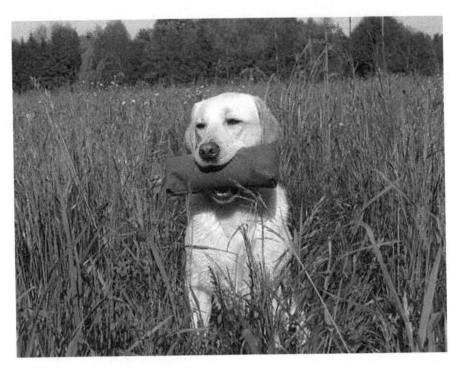

What are the Roles that Psychiatric Service Dogs play in the Lives of a Disabled Person?

A disabled person that has a psychiatric disability which limits their access to living a fulfilled life can be better served by having a Psychiatric Service Dog as a companion. This can open up doors for them that they never imagined and allow them to experience life without limitations. Psychiatric Service Dogs are specifically trained to perform tasks that allow this to happen.

As a Psychiatric Service Dog, the training can be intense and specific to their handler's needs. They must adhere to a higher standard of training and be able to handle many more things with diplomacy. For instance, a Psychiatric Service Dog needs to be able to enter a crowded area without being bothered by other animals or people. This is something that they must be trained to do. Most dogs will not handle other animals in their space easily. However, as a Psychiatric Service Dog, they need to act as if that other animal is not even there. Psychiatric Service Dogs provide such services listed below:

- Answering the door for their handler if they are unable to do that. They do this by pulling a lever or, if the house is fitted specifically for this service, by applying pressure to a part of the door where it can be opened.

- Picking things up and bringing them to the handler, such as medication, something they dropped or the mail.

- Alerts others to the handler in times of extra assistance from a caretaker. This is a way of alerting the nurse or caretaker that the disabled person needs their services.

- Provides mobility support as well as the ability to climb stairs, get up off of furniture, and navigate tight areas or areas with limited visibility. This is done by leading the handler with a strong lead or leash. This can help them when out in public or at home.

- Providing stability and support for those that have imbalance issues is another way that a Psychiatric Service Dog can help their handler. Many dogs provide this service for those that are arthritic, have equilibrium issues or even stroke victims.

- Provides a saddle bag for the handler and carries medicine, diabetic supplies, anxiety supplies, and such. This allows the handler to have access to leaving their home without having to worry about carrying their medical needs with them.

Psychiatric Service Dogs can also provide services for their handlers in times of emergency, such as:

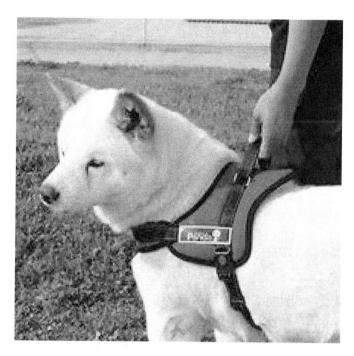

- Retrieves the phone for the handler when they need to contact 911 or a family member for help, as well as pushing an alert button when the handler needs service.

- Barks into the speakerphone for emergency services to know that the handler is either in danger or needs emergency services. This is a way for the emergency services to know that the person in need is not only disabled but also in need of assistance.

- Responds to the handler in appropriate ways to interrupt or alert them to a psychiatric episode or occurrence. This helps the handler know that an episode is coming or helps pull them out of an episode that could potentially cause them more pain or struggle.

- Provides an alarm for the handler when they are having an episode or in distress so that other people will be aware of the episode. This allows them to get help for their handler and provide the necessary medical treatment that their handler needs.

- When experiencing a seizure or anxiety episode, they will alert others to you and bring them over, so they can assist you in your needs. This works great for when you are down on the floor with an episode, seizure or suicide attempt. This is especially helpful for those that suffer from severe depression, mood disorders, anxiety, and seizures.

- Uses a system to alert the handler and the fire department or neighbors to a fire, burglary or other issues that would require the handler to evacuate the home or call the police.

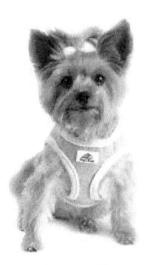

These are all the services that allow the handler or disabled person the ability to live their lives without fear of what would happen during these situations. These are just a few of the services that can be provided by a Psychiatric Service Dog. There are so many ways that a Psychiatric Service Dog can modify or help a disabled person's life. With a Psychiatric Service Dog, the disabled person is able to feel more confident in themselves and their abilities to live alone or explore their towns or take a vacation without needing a constant caretaker or nurse on call.

- As a Psychiatric Service Dog, their role is to provide the disabled handler with the freedoms and luxuries that others get to enjoy.

- They help to aid them with episodes of disassociation with the surrounding area. They also provide the handler with the ability to have stability when they are disoriented due to medications.

- They can provide the handler with an alert that will inform them that it is time to take medication.

- Often times, when people are having anxiety, panic attacks or episodes, they need tactile stimulation that will bring them out of those episodes or help them be aware of when the episode is coming on. The Psychiatric Service Dog is trained to provide these services.

- They are also trained to recognize when someone is hallucinating and how to handle them when they come.

- For those handlers that are experiencing PTSD from being attacked or being at war, they can benefit from having a Psychiatric Service Dog. This dog can provide them with someone that checks every room before they enter and alert them if everything is okay or not in the room.

- If someone has the potential to self-harm or has self-harmed in the past, then a Psychiatric Service Dog will provide them with interruption to these behaviors. This will help those that are OCD about these behaviors.

With all these services that a Psychiatric Service Dog can provide, you can see the benefits that they could give to the lives of disabled people. Many U. S. Veterans are looking for assistance in medical stabilization after returning from war, and a Psychiatric Service Dog can be the key to providing them the stability in their medical treatment that they need outside of medication and counseling.

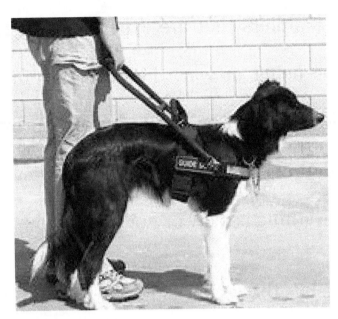

By caring for a Psychiatric Service Dog, it provides them the necessary reasons to take care of themselves and another living with them. This, oftentimes, can provide them with a purpose and a means for leaving their house. This allows the opportunity to go outside and have interactions with others, as well as provide them with a reason for leaving their comfort zone and experiencing more things in life.

When people with depression think of leaving their homes, they are not too thrilled about the idea. Having a Psychiatric Service Dog will provide them with a reason to get out of bed and get fresh air. Fresh air and sunlight provide Vitamin D, which is a vital nutrient that is needed for us to be happy and can increase our moods. Fresh air has been known to reverse the effects of depression as well as the symptoms that depressed people experience. This is also something that can be provided to a handler through an Emotional Support Animal. Through scientific and clinical studies, people with disabilities have expressed a greater rate of self-esteem, independence as well as happiness when living with a service animal or emotional support animal.

One dog is capable of helping over 60 people. Through programs that allow Veterans to train a Psychiatric Service Dog, they not only train the dog how to serve but heal themselves by giving them a purpose. This helps them cope with PTSD and other issues. They help reduce the anxiety of the handler so that they can sleep better, which in turn helps them improve their health. By training the dog to experience new environments, the handler is, in turn, bringing themselves out of the isolation that many people who suffer

PTSD or depression will place themselves in. When the veterans train the dog that they can trust the world and that it is a safe spot to be in, they are also learning this lesson themselves.

Psychiatric Service Dogs provide a boost of confidence for children as well as adults that suffer from Psychiatric disorders. There have been several research studies that have proven that a Psychiatric Service Dog helps release the dopamine levels or oxytocin levels within the handler. These two levels are related to stabilizing the moods and helping the wellbeing of the handler. Children who have confidence issues or autism can use a Psychiatric Service Dog to feel more confident when having to engage with other people. It teaches them to interact with the dog, which helps them to learn how to interact with other people.

Although the training for a Psychiatric Service Dog can be super specific and intense, the benefit far outweighs the expense of time or money that is put into it. It can take weeks to months to train a Psychiatric Service Dog depending on the training that is needed and the dog's ability to adapt to the tasks that are being asked of them—but do not fear. This is something you can do yourself by applying the techniques in this book.

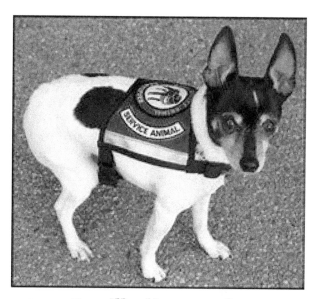

In the next chapter, I will discuss the necessary skills that are needed to become a Psychiatric Service Dog and how to ensure that your dog will have these skills. The rest of this book will focus on choosing the right dog for the task as well as the choice of equipment for your dog to adapt to your needs. I will also discuss the laws that regulate what you can and cannot do with your Psychiatric Service Dog and the necessary role your dog must play when out in public. The last part of this book will focus on training techniques for specific services that your Psychiatric

Service Dog will need to be able to perform for your needs.

Like what you're reading? Want to hear this as an audio book? Click here to get this book for FREE when you join Audible!!

https://adbl.co/2YqyNOh

CHAPTER 2: WHAT ARE THE NECESSARY SKILLS NEEDED TO BE A PSYCHIATRIC SERVICE DOG?

There are a few necessary skills that your dog must have to be a Psychiatric Service Dog. Each one of these skills is to ensure that your dog is being of service to you in the best feasible way. Each skill set is used to determine if this is the right dog for your needs and if they are able to acquire the training that is necessary for you.

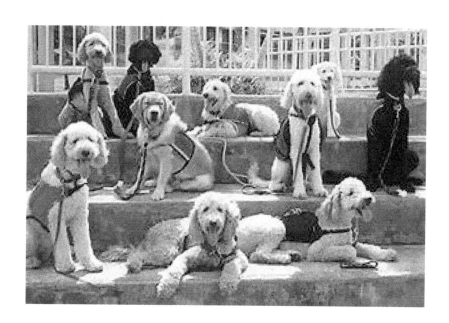

In order for a dog to be a viable choice for a Psychiatric Service Dog, they must exhibit what some people call the Good Companion Training. With Good Companion Training, your dog will learn how to be obedient to you. Since every dog is different, this can mean different things for each dog. A dog with this training will not jump on others, bark or growl when not appropriate, not dig in the yard, or climb on the furniture if you do not want them to. They will not chew on something they are not supposed to or bite others. They will not eat off others' plates or snatch things out of babies' hands. These are considered basic obedience training steps. A few of the things that are involved with basic obedience are listed below.

- Being able to heel or slow their pace when the handler has slowed, stopped, or made a certain sound or movement, as well as they heel when released off the leash when given a specific command and not resume walking until told to.

- Another skill is being able to stand perfectly still while the vet or handler examines the dog for a check-up. Sometimes, we need to examine our pets to see if something is bothering them, or the vet needs them to be still for exams. This is a necessary skill to have.

- When the handler has released the Psychiatric Service Dog from the leash, the dog needs to be able to stay close to the handler and return to the handler with a simple command if sent to retrieve something.

- Another obedience skill that the dog needs to have is to be able to sit for over 1 minute without moving from the spot. This is to ensure that the dog can follow the command of sit and stay.

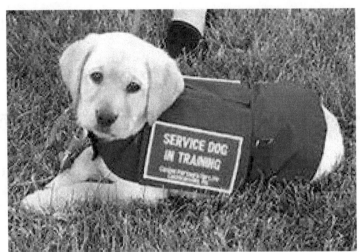

- Along the same lines of sit and stay is the down and stay skill that is also necessary for a Psychiatric Service Dog. When out in public, your Psychiatric Service Dog needs to be able to sit for over 3 minutes while you eat, change clothes, check out at the register, use the restroom, and much more. They must be able to stay without getting up or losing focus.

- Dropping something or giving something to you on command is an important part of obedience skills. Being able to command your dog to drop it or give it to you can mean the difference between a Psychiatric Service Dog that collects things and brings them to you and one that does not.

- Another obedience skill that is useful to have is to be able to follow hand signals without voice commands. Some disabled people cannot speak, and this can be confusing for a dog that has learned with auditory commands. In this instance, the Psychiatric Service dog would need to be able to respond to hand signals instead of auditory signals.

- Another thing that a dog should learn is to retrieve and return. This means that the dog should be able to leave the handler, retrieve something that was dropped or needed from a distance and return the item to the handler.

- The dog should also be able to ignore sudden loud or strange noises that can arise. When a dog startles easily with noise or strange sounds, this can be a problem. The Psychiatric Service Dog should not alert or respond to anything that the handler has not said or done.

- Another thing that goes along with this is that they should be able to walk on unfamiliar surfaces without being uncomfortable. Often times, a new surface will startle a dog or create anxiety about being on it. The Psychiatric Service Dog should be comfortable approaching or walking on any surface it comes in contact with.

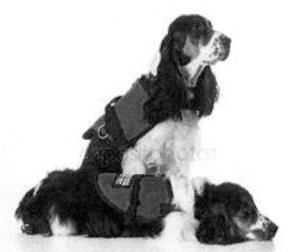

- Psychiatric Service Dogs should be comfortable around people who have canes, wheelchairs, children, strangers, and also those that create loud noises like the mentally-challenged individuals. They should not respond to other people but instead act as if they are not there unless told by the owner that it is ok.

- Another part of this would be not alerting to other animals. Since dogs tend to chase cats and small prey or respond to other dogs with interest or disgust, a Psychiatric Service Dog should respond as if the other animals are not there. This ensures that they are focused on their handlers' needs instead of losing focus and being distracted.

A great starting point for a dog that is intended to be a Psychiatric Service Dog is to enroll them in the Canine Good Citizen training course. This course is taught to ensure that the dog is a good citizen, and it is also a jumping off point to ensure that your choice of Psychiatric Service dog was best suited to you. It trains the dog how to be well-mannered with the other animals, people, and specific situations. Since this is a training course that provides certification through the American Kennel Club and its approved trainers, this is something that will need to be done by someone certified to teach the course. However, if you adopt a dog from the shelter, often times they will be provided with this training, and it will be included in their bio and their adoption fee.

Some of the training that is provided in this course can include:

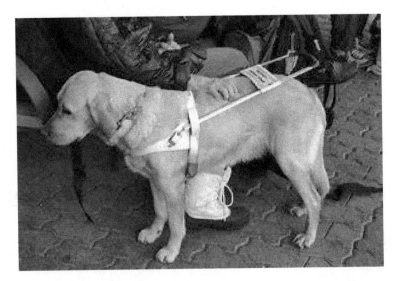

• Allowing a friendly stranger to approach them and communicate with them.

• Sitting in a polite manner while someone pets them.

• Allowing someone to groom them without aggravation and also check on their extremities.

• Walking beside their owners with a loose leash without pulling or bolting.

- Passing through a crowd without being bothered by other people or animals.

- Sitting and laying on command and staying for a length of time that the handler decides.

- Coming to the handler when they are called from a distance of 10 feet.

- Showing no reaction or only positive reactions to another dog.

- Responding appropriately to a distraction that is provided by the trainer.

- Staying for extended periods of time without the handler in a supervised separation. This ensures that the dog will not have separation anxiety.

Another crucial factor is that they should have skills that fit within your choice of lifestyle. Often times, a depressed person will spend hours in bed, sometimes even days. The Psychiatric Service Dog that you choose should be able to not potty in the house for the long hours that the handler is in bed, as well as motivate the handler to exit their bed and take them outside for potty times.

CHAPTER 3: HOW TO PICK THE RIGHT PSYCHIATRIC SERVICE DOG

By starting off with knowing exactly what you are expecting from your Psychiatric Service Dog, you can begin to find the right dog that is suited for your needs. In order to know exactly what you will need you, should simply ask yourself a few questions.

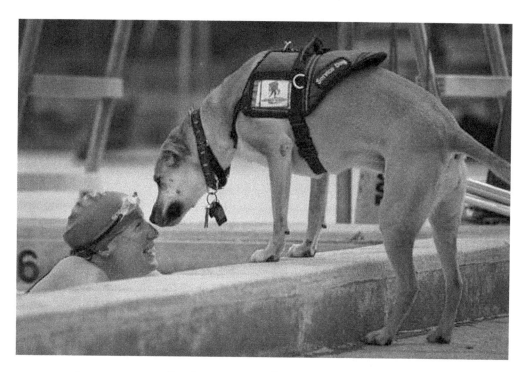

These questions can help you determine your needs and the appropriate dog that will fit these needs. You should also determine what your limitations will be in caring for your chosen Psychiatric Service Dog.

You will need to start with making a list of your Psychiatric Service Dog needs. Ask yourself these questions:

- What will your Psychiatric Service dog do for you?

- How will you train your Psychiatric Service dog to do the tasks that you need?

Next, list the disabilities that you will need assistance from the Psychiatric Service dog for.

- Do they need to react to what you react to?

- Do they need to be non-reactive?

- Do they need to assist you in not engaging in a destructive behavior?

- Do you want a redirect or a complete stop of the behavior?

- Is there a physical manifestation that will help your dog recognize the issue?

- Is the interaction with the dog needed to change your physiology?

- Is there another way that the Psychiatric Service Dog can assist you with these issues?

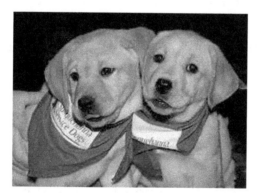

Next, you will need to discuss with your doctor or those that are closest to you to determine if they have any ideas or actions that need to be curtailed or stopped. Discuss how your disability has interfered with or impacted your life, and if there is something that would be beneficial to what your Psychiatric Service Dog could help with. Discuss with others that own a Psychiatric Service Dog and find out how theirs is helping them in their life or making their life more manageable. Ask if there is something specific that they trained their Psychiatric Service Dog to do that would also benefit you. Then create a list of the things that you will need your Psychiatric Service Dog to do for you to assist you in living a more comfortable life.

Once you get to this point, you will need to specify the size of the breed of dog that you will use. For instance, a dog for balance will need to be large. An average-sized person needs a dog weighing at least 50 pounds for him to be stable. For a larger size person, you may need a bigger dog for stability. If the need is not associated with stability, then a smaller breed dog will be a good option. They need less space in your home, their food intake is minimal, and since they live longer life spans, they will provide you with a longer Psychiatric Service Dog time period. They are a great asset for tactile stimulation and also alerting for behavior modification or episodes.

The next thing that you will need to think of is the personality that you have and the dog's personality. Will you mesh well with specific breeds more than others? If you are thinking of a dog that is naturally inclined to chase down vermin, then they will be more independent than those that are used for retrieving the game that is shot down. A dog breed that is assigned to be guard dogs will need to be handled by someone that is confident with their handling abilities, which means that they would not be an excellent choice for a Psychiatric Service Dog. A toy breed dog is an excellent dog for companionships and Psychiatric Service dogs.

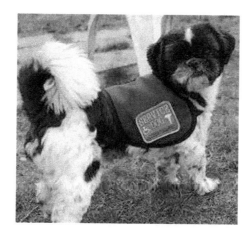

Talk to a professional trainer that is specialized in choosing the appropriate dog for a Psychiatric Service Dog based on the needs of the handler and see what they suggest for your needs. The trainer does not have to be a trainer for a Psychiatric Service Dog. Any trainer that works with dogs that are trained for agility, competition trainers, sports trainers, as well as search and rescue trainers can be a valuable resource to finding out information on specific breeds that will help you.

Another source of identifying the right breed for your needs is to contact other people who have trained their own Psychiatric service dogs. Get insight on how they chose their dog breed and the methods they used to identify the appropriate breed for their needs.

Now, you should consider your activities every day. Are you active or inactive? A dog will need to have at least one walk a day to explore the world, sniff out the other dogs in the area, and enjoy nature. A Psychiatric Service Dog has needs that are not easily ignored. They will need to potty and have exercise. A family member is an excellent source of getting help with your Psychiatric Service Dog. However, the goal should be for you to get outside and experience the world. There are also several services that will come to your home and walk your dog for you for a fee.

If you do not like lots of activity, then you need to choose a dog that has low-energy levels, such as a Shih Tzus or another small dog. A medium energy style dog will need at least one hour or more of continuous exercise each day. This can be a Labrador Retriever or something similar. If you find that a higher energy breed dog is a good option for you, then choose something like a Border Collie or even a Boxer. These types of dogs will need to run for a length of time for at least 1 to 2 hours per day. They thrive within dog sports type of activities and need constant activity to keep busy.

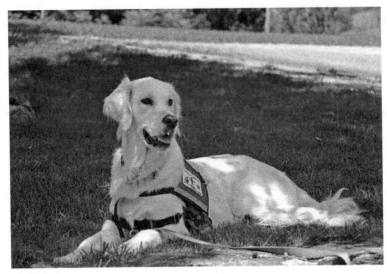

If you do not have a lot of active days, then do not try to overestimate the activity within your life. This can only mean disaster or destructive behaviors that can come from boredom. A dog with minimal energy can be over-exercised. However, a dog with extra energy with minimal exercise is going to be disastrous in the long run.

If you enjoyed an active lifestyle prior to your disability, such as agility, flyball, dancing, or any other physical stimulation, then choosing a dog that is active in moderation can be a great option as your Psychiatric Service Dog. This will also help you to get outside and be active, giving you back your previous lifestyle prior to the disability.

Second to last, you will need to consider the grooming required for the dog. Although grooming can be a very therapeutic activity, it is also something that people with arthritis will have struggles with. It does provide a repetitive behavior for someone who finds that they are OCD about actions to have an alternative to replace those behaviors with.

However, there are certain conditions that can be affected severely by the presence of hair or the need to groom a dog. Someone who is in a depressive state may find themselves lethargic and unable to care for the dog's grooming. This can present a problem for the dog's hair and health. On the same note, someone who is OCD about germs and cleanliness may find that a dog's hair or grooming a dog to be overwhelming and disgusting. This can actually create more anxiety in the situation.

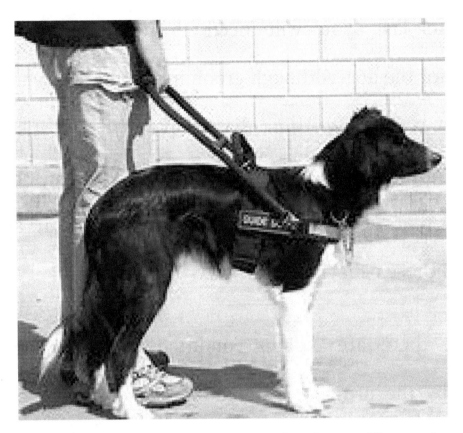

By deciding what will bother you and what will not bother you with regards to your dog's grooming, you can be better prepared for the necessary upkeep and maintenance. Although every person with the same diagnosis is different, the grooming of a dog is specific to each breed. A long-haired dog will need the same grooming procedures as another long-hair dog will need. So, determine what it is that you are willing to do on a daily basis for your Psychiatric Service Dog before picking the breed that you will use.

A Greyhound or a Pit Bull has a short coat that is smooth and sheds minimally. They do not require copious amounts of grooming. Dogs such as Golden Retrievers, German Shepherds, as well as a Labrador Retriever can have a coat that is either short or medium in length. They tend to shed often and need to be copiously brushed 3 times per week.

A long-coated dog such as a Lhasa Apso as well as a Blue Heeler will need to be brushed often. This will need to be done every day. They will also need a regular grooming appointment at the dog salon to get a haircut. If you have allergies, then the Poodle, Schnauzer, and Bichon Frise will need to be your optimal choice. They do not shed and are hypoallergenic. They will need regular grooming with brushes or combs. They should be groomed every 2 days and have a regular haircut. A mixed breed dog can be quite different and difficult to gauge when it comes to shedding and grooming needs. They will have needs based on the mixture that is in them.

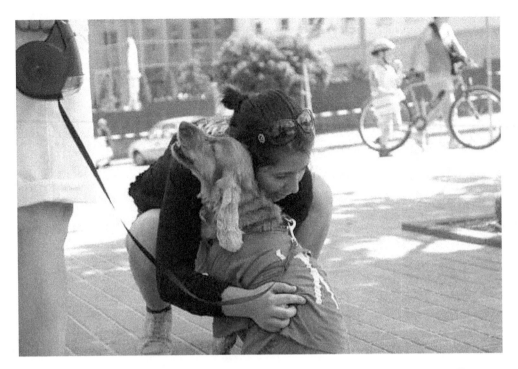

Finally, consider your work or home life schedule and as well as the tasks that you are already responsible for. Think about the other people in your life. Think about your home life. Think about your work environment or doctors' offices that you visit. Ask yourself these questions:

- Are they allergic to dogs?

- Do you live in a colder climate or a hotter climate?

- Do you visit places that require a quiet environment?

- Will it be troublesome to carry a cloth to always wipe up slobber?

- Do you live in a small apartment in a big city?

- Are you traveling on planes or trains often?

Now, add up all the answers you received from the questions and find the right dog for you.

Do some research on the dog breeds that meet your needs and begin compiling the pros and cons on which breed is the best one for you. Once you have narrowed it down, go to some breeders and shelters and get a feel for the dog, its mentality, and connection with its handler.

Which dog is best for you and your needs?
Some dogs are specifically bred for their mentality. These dogs would make great Psychiatric Service Dogs.

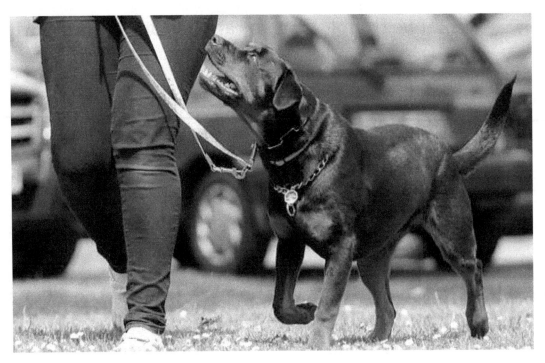

If the person that is handling the dog does not have the ability to brush their own hair, then they should not have a dog that will require copious amounts of grooming. Dogs that require copious amounts of care should only be considered for those handlers that need the motivation to be active in life. For those that need a reassuring and gentle breed, then choosing a dog that is bred for those qualities should be the most important first step.

There are several breeds of dog in the world that would qualify for a Psychiatric Service Dog. These can be anything from a Chihuahua to a Pitbull. Any dog is an acceptable option. However, some dogs that have a specific need would require more time and energy to maintain than others. Knowing what you are needing and looking for is going to be the determining factor in picking the perfect dog.

Below, I will give specific natural qualities to several of the dog breeds that people have been using for Psychiatric Service dogs in the past 10 years. This will give you a base to rate your perfect dog by.

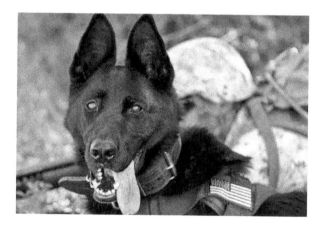

Some of the most people-pleasing dog breeds are:

- Beagles

- Cavalier King Charles Spaniel

- Flat-coated Retriever

- Collie

- Pug

- Irish Setter

- French Bulldog

- Bichon Frise

- Bulldog

- Maltese

Dogs that are great for a small to medium-sized house:

- Toy Poodle

- Cavalier King Charles Spaniel

- Pug

- Bichon Frise

- Yorkshire Terrier

- Corgi

- Dachshund

- French Bulldog

- Beagle

- Chihuahua

Dogs that fall under the general area of acceptable Psychiatric Service Dogs:

- Labrador Retriever

- Beagle

- Rottweiler

- Saint Bernard

- Pomeranian

- Standard Poodle

- French Bulldog

- Pug

- Greyhound

- German Shepherd

- Golden Retriever

With all the different breeds that we have listed here, I want to give you some insight into how several of these dogs will provide adequate, if not excellent, help as a Psychiatric Service Dog. To start off, I will discuss the Standard Poodle.

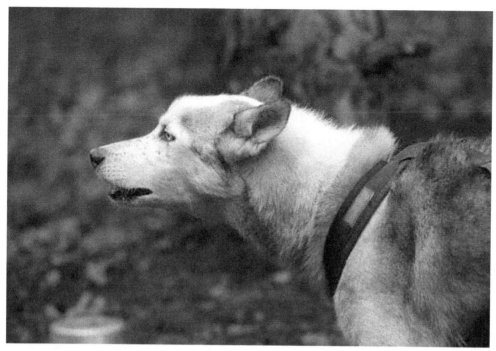

The Standard Poodle

These dogs are very bright and are easily trainable. They have an exceptional ability to pick up quickly on training commands and are especially eager to please the handler. Poodles are widely liked due to their brilliant minds. Because of their original breeding training of retrieval, they have the tenacity for following cues that are given by their handlers for helping those that need someone to pick up and retrieve items for them.

Another positive for poodles as Psychiatric Service Dogs is that they have a low shed ratio compared to other dog breeds. The low shedding also means that they have a hypoallergenic coat making them an excellent choice for those with allergies to pets and pet dander.

The Poodle is an affectionate dog that is good-natured, especially with children and disabled individuals. They have been known to excel in obedience training courses and are loyal to their handlers. They are great for those that suffer from depression, anxiety, as well as panic attacks. Since Poodles notice the moods of their handlers, they can know indirectly that their handler is unhappy. This is something that does not have to be taught to them; they are naturally sensitive. After the proper training techniques are taught, they can become attuned deeply to the handler's moods and have a connection to their handler that can help them identify and divert the handler from self-destructive behaviors.

The Havanese

Although the Havanese is a small pooch, they have a highly intelligent characteristic. This allows them to be trainable, making them a suitable selection for Psychiatric Service Dog. They have a friendly personality that helps them be a great family pet choice as well as a great option for children with disabilities. The Havanese is an excellent choice for those that are suffering from depression due to their friendly personalities. They are also outgoing, showering their handler with love and cuddles, which can improve the person's disposition. They thrive on love and enjoy snuggles with their handler. This means that they will be a great companion for someone that suffers from mood disorders.

Because of their sensitivity, they are able to attune themselves to their handler's emotional energy. This allows them to know when their handler is having an emotional episode, and they need support or comfort. This also makes them loyal and a great dog for your lap when you need comfort.

They know tricks such as retrieving medications for their owners as well as interrupting the behaviors that can be harmful or repetitive and can be self-destructive. By providing a focal point, a child with Autism is able to bring both the autistic world together with the real world.

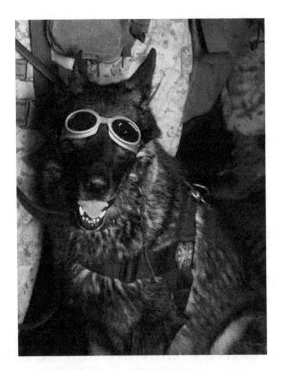

The Cavalier King Charles Spaniel

They have an enormous personality that makes them very friendly and lovable. They enjoy snuggling and showing affection to their handlers as well as others. They bond strongly with their handler as well as the children within their household. This is where they get the name "Velcro pooch." Because of this, they are an amazing Psychiatric Service Dog for those that suffer from PTSD and depression.

While petting a King Charles Spaniel, the repetition will help create tranquility and calm within their mind. This helps tremendously with those that need a calming activity to help them deal with their disabilities. Cavaliers are not at all aggressive towards people and children. This means that they are a great option for those that need a Psychiatric Service Dog who can be in public without being aggressive to other people and animals. They do need lots of training prior to being used when in public, though. However, this dog's intelligence makes it super easy for them to learn their necessary training commands.

The Cavalier is a very gentle, quiet breed, which makes them an excellent breed for PTSD handlers as well as those that suffer from anxiety. They are intuitively linked to their handlers, making it easier for them to identify with the handler and connect with all of their emotional episodes.

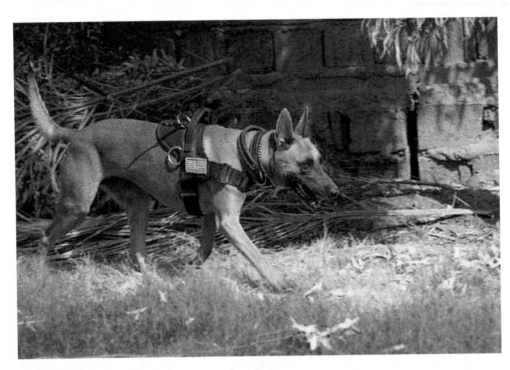

The Labrador Retriever

The Labrador Retriever has a superior intelligence to other dogs. This makes them an excellent choice for not only Psychiatric Service Dogs but also as great companion animals. They also tend to be very gentle towards their handlers and children.

Since the retriever was originally bred for retrieving, this means they make an excellent Psychiatric Service Dog for those that need help retrieving their mail, as well as picking things up that they have dropped. This shows how their intelligence, eagerness to please, and obedience provide them the capabilities of being a Psychiatric Service dog.

They maintain a stable and balanced personality, which helps tremendously with ADHD and ADD children and adults. This also provides them with the necessary temperament for Autistic children and adults. They help the Autistic handler to be calmer and more settled during moments of outbursts. Individuals that are suffering from schizophrenia will also feel safer and secure due to the ability to focus on the care of their dog and the calmness that these dogs provide to the environment.

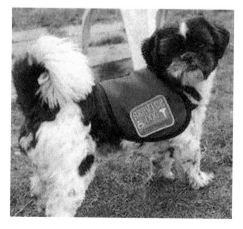

The Miniature Schnauzer

Yet another small breed dog that makes an excellent choice for a Psychiatric Service Dog. This miniature dog is a spirited dog with lots of spunk. They love to romp and play. But they also love to lay and be cuddled. They make a great sidekick for those that need to be more active in life or those that love to be active but need to have the Psychiatric support that the Psychiatric Service Dog will provide.

They have a high intelligence level and learn how to be obedient and a people pleaser fairly easily. They pick-up on social and emotional cues which makes them a great companion for those with emotional instability.

The German Shepherd

Although most people think these dogs make superb police dogs, they do not realize that they can make excellent Psychiatric Support or Psychiatric Service Dogs as well. The German Shepherd is a very tenacious and smart dog breed with the discipline to learn all they are taught. They are eager to please their handlers and love to show affection. They perform remarkably when asked to, and this is no different when the disabled person needs help from them. This can make them a great asset for handlers that have mental health issues.

Because of all the natural character traits of the German Shepherd, they make an excellent choice for those suffering from OCD symptoms as well as anxiety issues. If trained properly, they will be able to detect when their handler is having a panic attack or onset of a panic attack and then prevent the panic attack from coming on. They can be trained to interrupt the behaviors with a pawing technique that will redirect the handler to a new behavior or action.

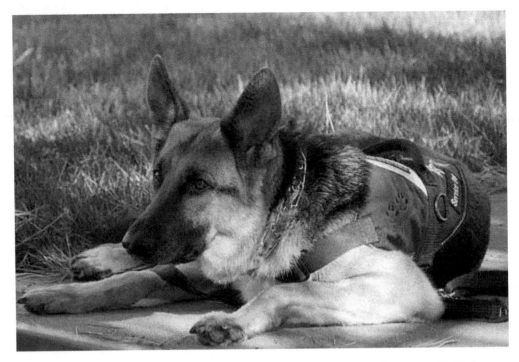

The gentleness of the breed and the loyalty they exhibit towards their handlers makes them a great dog for PTSD sufferers. They are an excellent choice for searching homes for any signs of unsafe people or activities. They are easy to train due to their ability to process knowledge quickly and have a similar intelligence level to humans. They provide a calming environment and can be depended on for moral support as well as provide safety.

The Lhasa Apso

The Lhasa Apso is a breed that has natural instincts that alert people of intruders. This means they make great Psychiatric

Service Dogs for those that need an alert dog for specific triggers or behaviors. They will make great companions as well as Psychiatric Service Dogs for those dealing with PTSD, as well as bipolar disorder and depression.

They have a cheerful disposition and will put a smile on anyone's face. This makes them a great option for calming and cheering up those that are depressed. They also have an uncanny knack for helping identify the different moods that their handler will display during a bipolar episode, and through training, they can learn how to react in an appropriate manner, such as nudging the handler to alert them of the change in moods. This will place the handler back on course for the right mood.

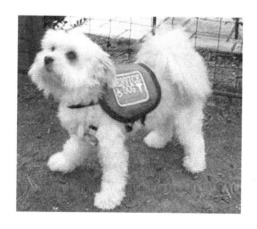

They tend to be comical and entertaining, which helps them uplift the morale of those that are depressed or bipolar. This makes them an excellent source of companionship with those that deal with mood disabilities.

Now that I have given you a few insights into how to pick a good Psychiatric Service Dog, the rest of this chapter will assist you in whether you should get a shelter dog or a pure breed dog, and if you should start with a puppy or an adult dog.

Shelter dog vs. pure breed dog

Shelter dogs come in all shapes and sizes. Some of the dogs that

you can find within the shelter are, believe it or not, actually purebred dogs that have been left by their owners due to housing or financial circumstances. So, what you might find out about shelter dogs is that they can actually be pure-bred dogs, as well as mutts.

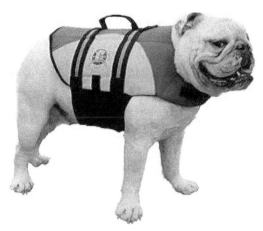

Breeders are able to provide you with a medical history and family bloodline for the dog that you are considering using as a Psychiatric Service Dog. This information can be useful for not only the genetic history of the dog but also for the personal information so that you will know if the temperament is ideal for your needs. When you examine the bloodline of the dog that you are choosing, you will be aware of any genetic medical issues that can affect your dog. This helps you know if the dog breed that you are choosing will have continuous issues with their hips or other genetic issues. Within dogs, personalities are inherited and passed down. This can be troublesome when picking out a shelter dog since you do not have any genetic background or know the parents of the dog that you are picking out.

If the background of the dog's family tree is riddled with Psychiatric Service dogs, genetically, the dog will be an excellent choice for a Psychiatric Service dog as well. If y o u need a dog that provides stability, then you will need to ensure that your Psychiatric Service Dog does not have a predisposition for hip dysplasia or joint pains. Running a genetic test will help you to know these details about the dogs that you are choosing between.

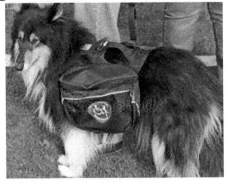

A breeder will charge more for a dog that is a purebred with a great genetic background. Although this can be expensive from the beginning, it can end up costing you much less in the long run. Especially if you have obtained a shelter dog that needs 2 hip replacements.

Although a rescue or shelter dog may seem like a great idea in the beginning, they can cost more money in the long run if they have health conditions that need to be maintained. They can also become bonded too intensely to their new owners and this can create separation anxiety, which can be exceedingly difficult to deal with. Rescue centers and shelters offer a very inexpensive way to obtain a dog that can be trained for Psychiatric Service Dogs. Most of the dogs that come from a shelter or rescue have already been fixed; they have had all their basic veterinarian needs to be met and have often times been tested for temperament as well as good citizenship. They are a much bigger risk in the genetic history and medical background since they are shelter or rescue pups.

A breakdown of how much a rescue or shelter dog and a pure-bred dog, can cost you is listed below for you to understand the difference in cost.

Rescued Adult already altered dog:

Adoption fee: $120

Veterinarian bills for genetic issues or health: $2000

Training cost of hiring out a trainer: $2000

Service Dog Gear: $100

Food and accessories: $1000

Grand Total: $5220

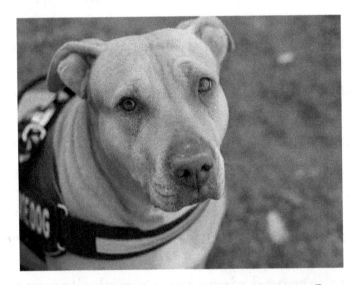

Dog Purchased from a Service Dog Breeder:

Purchase price: $2500

Veterinarian Bills: $750

Expenses for Training with a Trainer: $1100

Service Dog Gear: $100

Food and accessories: $1000

End Total: $5450

Even though the purchase price of a rescue or shelter dog is slightly less, the continued cost in the long run for medical expenses will drastically change this. The training cost will also be very different since, in the end, you will have to continuously train the shelter dog when new behaviors arise or to modify a negative behavior that will hinder your ability to train them at first. So, starting with a purebred dog from the beginning could only cost you the initial fees that are needed, instead of a continuous vet bill and retraining bill.

Remember that the dog you chose should be right for you and your needs. It should be as healthy as possible and have a lifespan that will give you the most benefit for the cost that you have put into it. You also need to remember that dogs that have unknown genetic backgrounds or are shelter dogs above the age of 3, can potentially have a reduced lifespan based on the genetic makeup as well as the amount of life left in them.

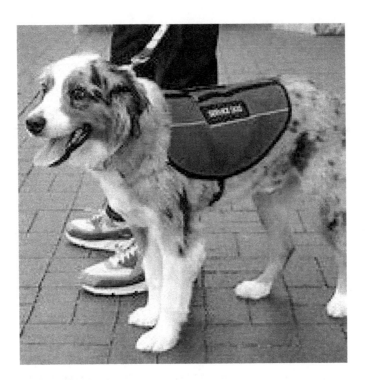

Puppy vs. Adult dog

Now that I have explained the differences between using a shelter dog versus a purebred dog you will be wondering if you need a pup or an adult. As with shelter or purebred dogs, you will need to decide based on your needs and what you want. A pup can be a wonderful experience if you are emotionally and physically ready to take care of a pup. However, if you are not, then you will need to get an adult dog. With a pup, you are able to watch as it grows and learns, seeing every milestone as they come around. With an adult, this has already taken place, and you may miss some of the fun and cute puppy stages. A puppy will also need to be trained in how to potty outside. This means lots of time spent crate training the new pup. Socialization is also necessary for a new pup as well. They will need to be introduced to other pups so they know how to play and not be aggressive toward other animals or people. Puppies tend to chew on everything, and training them not to chew can cost you time, money, and aggravation. Consider these when you are deciding on picking a pup or an adult dog.

Often times, you will find an adult dog is more stable in their personalities, and they are not in the chewing stages anymore. They tend to be well potty trained and know basic obedience. This gives them an advantage over a puppy, especially since puppies need all the extra work before they can start to be trained for Psychiatric Service Dogs. If you get a dog that is a retired show dog, you will have found a dog that is used to crowds and other animals. This means that the outside world will not be distracting to them. But this also means that as an adult, they may have 66 experienced situations in their lives that can create triggers or difficulties. This can make it harder for them to be trained, especially if they were traumatized at an early age by people or animals. Sometimes, the dog may be startled by someone coming up behind them and smacking them on the butt; this happens often. This can create a problem, especially if the dog bites the child due to past trauma. In the same instance, the dog could have had some negative experiences with men in hats and may respond in a negative way to a man in a hat. They may never learn how to be comfortable with those men. This can make it difficult to find a suitable adult dog that is a viable choice for your Psychiatric Service dog needs.

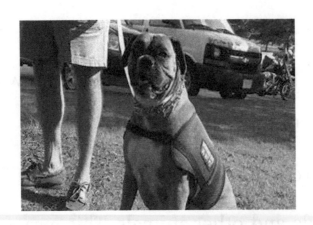

Another concern is the lifespan of the dog that you chose. That is why you should only start with a dog that is less than or no older than 2 years old.

There are several ways to test and see which dog is best for your needs. One way is to test their temperament. By testing the temperament of the dog, you are able to find out if the dog will be able to handle tricky situations. A great test to use for this type of testing is the Volhard Temperament Test.

Consider that an adult dog has a stable temperament when living in a stable home. An adult dog that is living in the shelter will be nervous and stressed. Therefore, the temperament of that dog is going to be hard to read at first. If the puppy has its temperament at 8 weeks, this cannot viably identify the temperament of the dog. The only thing that would be reliable would be the fear and confidence levels that are exhibited in new situations. Testing the mom of a puppy can give you the highest predictor of the puppy's ability to be a Psychiatric service dog. If the mom is a competent

Psychiatric Service dog with a great temperament, then the puppy will have a higher chance of being a great Psychiatric Service dog.

Due to all of this information, you should choose a pup that has a mother who is even and stable-tempered and is an acceptable Psychiatric Service dog or chose one that is living in a stable home with the right temperament. To find a puppy that is going to be the right temperament, you should find a Psychiatric Service dog breeder. The breeder can not only show you the temperament of the mother and father but also provide the family genetics of the pup. This will help you rule out any types of predispositions for genetic markers of disease and ailments. The mother is not required to be a Psychiatric Service dog for her to have a great temperament. Consider looking at dogs that are therapy dogs, dogs that have competency in obedience or service work, as well as extremely laid-back dispositions. Many of the dogs that are being bred for show-dogs are also being bred for the proper temperament for Psychiatric Service Dogs as well.

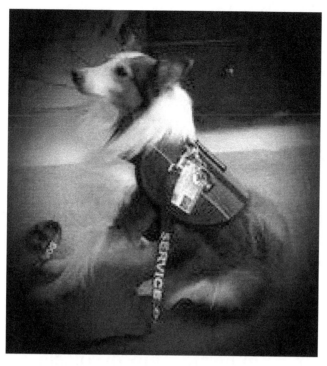

If you are interested in getting a suitable adult dog, then check into retired show-dogs. You will need a dog that has been living in a stable environment for an extended period of time. If you contact a breeder, you may be able to get a discount on a dog that has been returned or retired from being a show dog. When purchasing a dog that has been returned to the breeder, you are able to get one that is slightly cheaper as well as has a family history. Retired show-dogs have been extremely socialized. They are also trained by handlers that are experienced and knowledgeable.

The basic thing that you need to remember is that no matter which one you choose, whether breeder, rescue, pup or adult, you need to not worry about the cost of the dog since it will average out to be a great investment over the over-all lifetime of the dog. The cost of medical care or time that is wasted on a dog that unsuitable is far more important in the long run. Since the breeder puppy can cost $2000, and a hip replacement from an inherited hip dysplasia condition can cost twice if not more than that, you really need to consider finding a dog that has a family history along with it. A dog with emotional instabilities can cost $1000 to 2000 over the 20 private lessons that will be needed by the trainer.

So, although the puppy may be the cutest option, sometimes, it is best to go with an older dog so that you do not have to invest extra time and training into the puppy that has to obtain basic obedience, as well as potty training and chewing behaviors.

In the end, you are able to make the choice of whether you want to find your dog from the shelter or breeder and whether that dog will be a baby or an adult dog. It is all determined by how much money you want to spend in the long run over the lifetime of the dog.

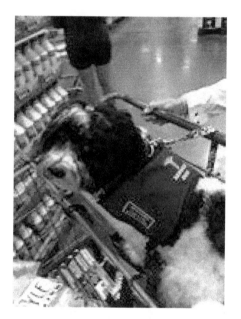

In the next chapter, you will learn about picking the right accessories and equipment that you will need for your Psychiatric Service Dog. I have given details about several types of collars and harnesses as well as leashes and how they benefit your training.

CHAPTER 4: PICKING THE RIGHT EQUIPMENT FOR YOUR DOG

Once you have located the exact dog that you will be using for your Psychiatric Service, you will need to determine what equipment as well as collars and leashes you will want to use. There are several options on the market today, and determining what you will use is based on your preference and needs.

A collar or harness has always been debated about within the dog owner's community. Several people believe strongly that a collar can cause choking, and they are right. However, your Psychiatric Service Dog should never be in a position that it would be choked by its collar. Many people believe that harnesses are the best for training and walking your dog. They feel that since it does not attach to the throat area, then it adds a safer way of keeping your dog under control. In this chapter, I will discuss the differences between the two and what you should consider making the deciding factor.

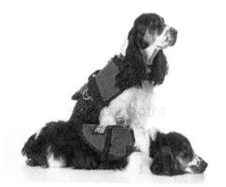

Collar vs. harness

What is the difference between a collar and a harness? Which one is the best for your dog? Which one will help you with the training process for a Psychiatric Service Dog? What will help you with your needs?

These are all questions that should be asked to help determine which one will provide you with the best options. There are some advantages to each one, and I will list below the different advantages.

- A harness is good for using when training a puppy that has not fully learned to walk. The harness can prevent the dog from getting tangled with the leash as well as hurting themselves.

- Harnesses provide more control for the handler. This is extremely important when training your dog on a busy street or large crowded area.

- When training an exceptionally large dog, you are able to have more control. This will also provide you the ability to take it easy on your back and arms.

- If a small dog pulls or tugs on a leash, they will be more easily able to get injured. Since the harness can help the pressure from the leash to be dispersed throughout the dog's body, this will lower the strain that is caused on the dog's back as well as the neck.

• A harness will also discourage the dogs from pulling. The harness can be attached to the dog's chest or shoulder blades. This will redirect the dog to not pull anymore since the pulling will not get him any results.

• Harnesses also provide a way for the dog to be confined to the leash without having the ability to escape the leash. Many dogs are little escape artists, and they will wiggle out of their collars and take off when not professionally trained. The harness prevents this from happening.

A few more pros about harnesses are listed below:

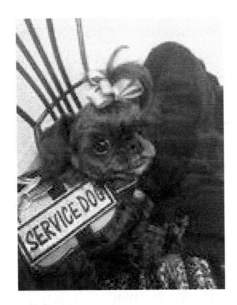

• They are an effective tool for training. This is especially true for puppies.

• A harness works well for most breeds, but specific breeds are highly benefited by wearing a harness. These dogs include pugs that are prone to having their eyeballs popping out due to pressure around their neck.

• They help you provide a more controlled pressure for the dog, which discourages them from pulling or tugging on the handler, as well as jumping.

• They will keep a distracted pup to focus extremely.

• A dog with a short nose is also a great candidate for using a harness. This is another reason a pug should be harnessed.

• If the dog has a neck injury or respiratory issues, then a harness will help with this. Due to the stress that a collar places on the throat when tugged, the windpipe can be aggravated, and this will cause coughing.

However, there are a few cons to using a harness. These will be listed below.

• Your dog may not be particularly fond of the harness.

• A harness that is clipped at the back will not be a complete success for your dog. The back-clip harnesses train the dog to focus their attention away from the handler, which is not a good thing.

Now, I will discuss the benefits of a collar for a dog in training. Below are the pros that can be derived about a collar when used for your dog in training.

- The can be a clever idea for the pups that dislike the harness and need that extra comfort.

- They are visible and function properly. They are able to provide a spot for your dog's identification, rabies tags, and license tag. This makes them convenient.

However, there are many cons with collars and your dogs. These can be located below.

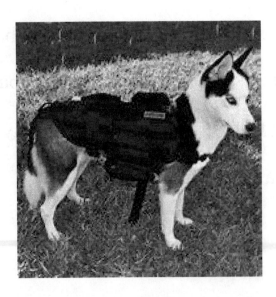

- They do not provide ideal training tools.

- If the dog pulls slightly, then it can increase the chances of an injury to the neck.

- The collar can cause pressure on the eye when they pull, and this can worsen the dog's progression of glaucoma or even increase signs of eye injuries.

- They can also increase the chances of thyroid problems as well as behavioral problems because of the increased pain and injuries to the ears and eyes due to the pressure on the neck.

As a precaution, a collar should be worn for identification purposes and harnesses for training and walking.

There are several varieties of harnesses and collars that can be purchased, each with a unique style and function. Below is a breakdown of the style of collars and harnesses that I have used in the past or have researched.

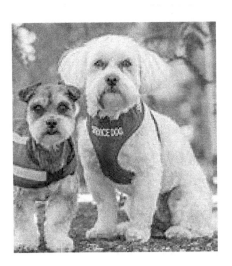

Flat Buckle Collar

The flat buckle collar is a popular one that many people use. This is mainly because it is basic and widely found. These are great for identification purposes. However, they do allow for the dog to pull and cause neck strain. If your dog is well-trained to walk on a leash and does not pull out of their collar, then this will do nicely.

Body Harness

Body harnesses are another extremely popular harness that is applied with a back attachment and is used most often with the small dog breeds. This harness is designed to prevent the throat from being damaged when the dog pulls on the leash. It also is quite helpful in keeping the leash from getting tangled underneath the dog's legs. The body harness will offer more control to the handler and less control to the dog. This will require you to have more control and strength. If you want to allow your dog to run and exercise, then the longer leash is ideal for this type of harness.

Easy Walk Harness

Easy Walk Harness has a leash attachment with a front facing harness. This can redirect the dog's attention away from pulling and also allow the handler to pull them back. The flexibility of the harness is a wonderful way to protect your dog that is sensitive to the neck, and it allows you to have 4 different adjustment points that can be a perfect fit for your dog.

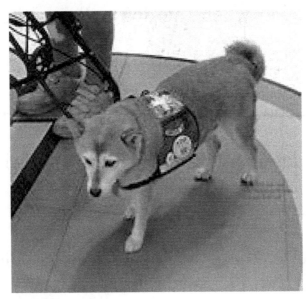

Soft Mesh Harness

Soft mesh harnesses are another wonderful way to get a

fashionable harness for your pet. They are lightweight and provide

a breathable harness for the dog. With the quick release

style buckle, you can easily adjust the harness. They come in

eight different brightly colored hues. These are a great option for

small dogs, especially the toy breeds. They are also a broad

selection for dogs that are sensitive around the neck and

puppies that need softer harnesses.

Nylon Dog Harness

Nylon dog harnesses are simple to adjust harness made of nylon

that can come in several sizes with fun colors to suit an

individual's personality. They can be priced very reasonably and suitable for all dogs.

Cooling and Reflective Harness

Harnesses with a cooling and reflective feature are another great option. They provide a cooling effect with a reflective quality. The cooling harness has a cooling pack that can be replaced for keeping the dog cool in the hotter months. Fill your pockets with some chilly water and place it in the freezer and this is guaranteed to keep the dog cool while doing agility and also hiking or hot weather walking.

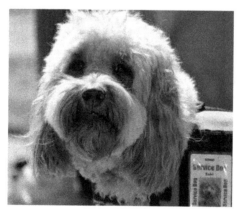

Front Hook Harness

A front hook harness looks similar to the body harness listed above, except the leash is attached in a different position which is on the front of the dog's chest area. This is a great harness for walking your dog since if the dog pulls, the harness will apply leverage and keep them from pulling.

Head Halters

Halters for the head are another way to apply a halter to your dog for control. This will provide you with all the control for your dog's head, and it keeps the dog in check and under control. This will give you the most opportunity for control when walking your dog. If you have an exceptionally large dog, then this is a great harness for you to use. It also provides leverage, which allows you to use less strength for the control. Using a long leash should never be done with a head halter. This can injure the dog if he pulls and is suddenly stopped by the leash.

Martingale Collars

Martingale collars are another collar that many people have been

using lately. Because of its ability to tighten around the neck of the dog, it has limited opportunity to slip off the dog's neck. The tightening only goes as far as the adjustment on the collar will allow. The traditional choke chain can cause lots of damage to the neck, so this collar was designed to not do the damage that the choke chain would do. However, it still provides the same function. Since dogs will wiggle out of their collars, this collar was designed to prevent that from happening. The leash is attached to a loop that is located on the collar, and this helps the collar tighten when needed.

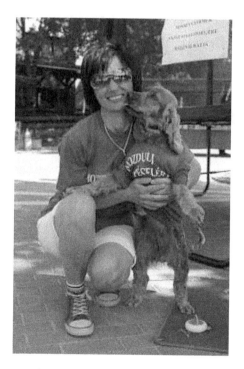

Leashes and the variety that you can choose from

Leashes are another accessory that is needed for training a dog for Psychiatric Services. Leashes come in several lengths as well as several styles. The leash that you chose is the most important piece of equipment for training your dog. A leash provides the handler with control as well as enforces the training procedures. By using the appropriate leash, you will help the dog to learn what is and is not acceptable behavior. In about every state, there is a leash law that states that a leash is required for pets and service animals. Leashes help to train your dog to behave properly. They also allow you to keep your dog safe and secure when outside.

Below, I have listed some of the most popular leashes on the market, and then I will go into a bit of detail about how they can help you with your needs.

- The Martingale leashes
- The Standard flat lead
- The Slip Leads
- The bungee and Stretchable rubber leashes
- The Retractable leashes

- The Gentle leader headcollar

- The Harness leads

The Martingale Leashes

The Martingale leash is similar in style to the Slip lead since they both function as a collar and a lead. This lead looks like a collar that is attached to a lead adding adjustability to the lead. This was designed for a smaller head and a thicker neck, such as Greyhounds. This means that it prevents the dog from backing out of the collar instead of being able to. It tightens on the dog to stop this behavior. These are not seen very often among dog trainers but can be used successfully with dogs that are prone to pulling. The martingale tightens to the strength at which it is being pulled. This leash also has an easy to attach and detach collar and leash. This means that it takes no time to put the lead on and off, so using it for a quick lead is a great idea.

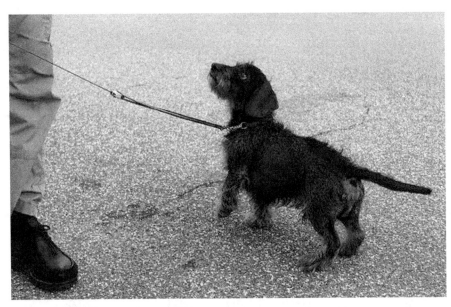

The Standard Flat Lead

This is the standard leash that everyone is using. They have a simple clamp or clasp that helps attach the leash to the collar or harness that is on the dog. They come in 4 foot or 8-foot lengths. They will clip onto the collar and allow your dog to have a range of walking space. The material options for a flat lead can be anything from nylon to leather. There are several styles, and the most popular ones are the ones that have a rope-like appearance. Since they are strong and excellent quality, they can work with any dog. They will provide a good bit of safety and allow the handler to have control of the dog. It is best to start off with a 4-foot leash so that you can be sure to have all the control. Once the dog is used to the procedures and has all the training they need, you can then extend your leash to a longer length. This is a staple in the accessories department of having a dog, even a Psychiatric Service Dog.

The Slip Leads

This is the leash style that is used at shelters. They function as both a collar and a leash. They are often used for training dogs since they are easily attached and detached from the dog's neck. They will look as if they are a regular leash, but they will have a small metal ring at the end of the leash. By pulling the leash through the metal ring, you can create a sort of collar to wrap around the dog's neck, creating a seamless leash and collar. The placement of this leash on a dog is especially important. It should be high up on the dog's neck closer to the ears so that it will not cause the dog to have any throat issues such as coughing or choking. This can be a sensitive area to the dog, so it will prevent the dog from pulling hard on the leash. This is not a long-term solution for dog training or safety.

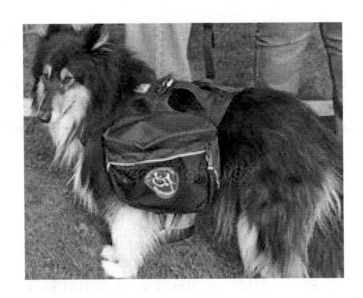

The Bungee and Stretchable Rubber Leashes

This is a leash that should be avoided at all costs. This does

not provide proper control for the handler when trying to correct

the dog's behaviors. Since the bungee or stretchable lead is

going to bounce back itself, this means that the handler is not

getting all the control they need to train the dog. This will

negate the ability of the handler to manage the dog.

The Retractable Leashes

A retractable leash is able to provide your dog up to 30 feet of

leash freedom. The leash is a thin braided rope that comes out of a

plastic handle. The handle contains a mechanical system that will

allow the leash to extend to full length, as well as a button that helps you retract the leash with a simple push of the button. It also provides a way to stop the leash from extending and retracting any further than a certain point. It is an extremely ineffective leash when needing a controlled environment. Since this does not have a quick response time, it allows the dog to get too far away and not provide enough control for the handler. This can lead to situations that can get extremely dangerous, especially if another dog confronts the dog. Another thing that is not effective with this leash is that the thin braided rope can get tangled up inside the mechanisms and be useless. It can also tangle up around the dog's legs and other extremities, as well as the hands of the owner. By using a retractable leash, you can influence your dog to believe that they are in control of you instead of you being in control of them. This does not give the dog clear boundaries and can be confusing to them.

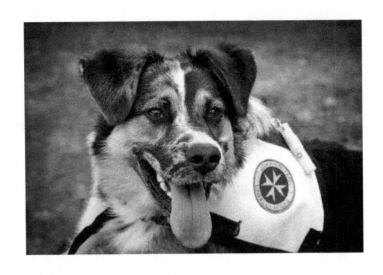

The Gentle Leader Headcollar

This is similar to a horse's muzzle and provides a gentler way to stop the pulling. This harness is slipped over the nose of the dog and used to pull the dog back to you with a gentle tug of the head towards you. This will redirect the dog's attention and give them a clear sign of who is in control. This, however, is an extremely uncomfortable leash for the dog. The dog's body language will give you a clue into how they feel about this type of harness and leash. If the dog shows signs of not liking it, then I would suggest not using it. The leash can cause hair loss around the muzzle as well as permanent indentions that can be uncomfortable for the dog. If you want a professionally trained dog, then this leash is not a great option since it just teaches them that you will jerk their head in the instance that they pull.

The Harness Leads

This is a lead and a harness that comes in one piece. This is usually used for dogs that jump. It is an effective way to teach them not to jump. The harness lead can tighten up around the dog's body when he tries to jump or pull. This harness will lessen the pressure that is applied to the trachea, and this is always a great option. However, making sure you use it properly is necessary to avoid the misuse of the leash and avoid the injuries that could ensue. On the other hand, using a traditional harness can provide too much pressure on the chest area, and this will result in the dog pulling much harder on the leash.

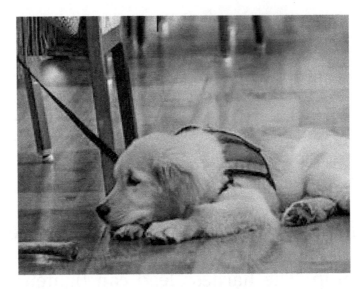

So, which leash is best for what type of dog and what should you chose seems to be the main question when it comes to leashes and your new Psychiatric Service Dog. If you have a hyper dog, you will need a leash that will allow you to control the dog. If the dog is not very hyper and tends to be laid back, then a leash that is looser in control will be a fine option for this type of dog. Every dog is different, and every leash provides a different amount of control as well as functionality.

Simple leash and collar

A simple leash with a collar can be an excellent choice for keeping a dog balanced and safe by your side. However, this is only best for the happy-go-lucky and calm dog. A dog with proper obedience training can be quite easily controlled with this leash.

Slip collar

If your dog presents issues while on a walk, a training lead can prove a great tool that offers a huge amount of control when the dog is misbehaving. This is a great collar and leash for a dog that gets easily distracted and can be a great asset for getting your dog's attention back to the task at hand. By giving a firm pull that is quick and to the side, you can divert the dog's attention back to the handler. This will knock the dog off balance and redirect his attention to the handler instead of the act of pulling. This will also allow you to keep the safety of your dog in mind, allowing you to give a safe correction to the dog.

CHAPTER 5: PET INSURANCE AND CARING FOR YOUR PSYCHIATRIC SERVICE DOG

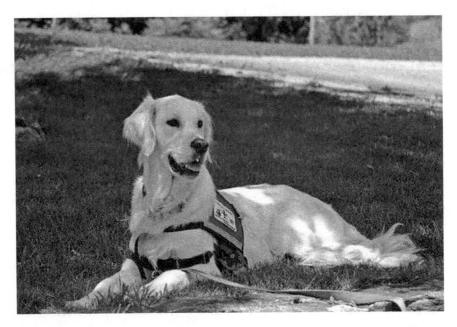

Another thing you will need to research as well as consider when looking to obtain or train your own Psychiatric Service Dog is the pet insurance and the amount of responsibility that you will have when caring for your dog.

Pet insurance is something that can be provided by a few service companies. There are also payment programs within veterinarian offices that provide you veterinarian services on a monthly payment basis. This is not a payment plan for services rendered but a plan that charges you per month for services yet to be rendered.

In this chapter, we will break down the benefits and advantages of owning a pet insurance plan, and the specific types that are available. I will also discuss the necessary services that your Psychiatric Service Dog will need to be fit as a fiddle. Then lastly, I will talk about how a wellness plan can differ from a pet insurance plan and what benefits you get from using one.

Pet Insurance vs. Wellness Plans with the Vet

Pet insurance is not like a traditional insurance plan for humans. If I was to go out and purchase an insurance plan for myself, it would cover routine check-ups and have a small coverage plan for the emergency services and surgeries. However, with a pet insurance plan, you will need to be covered for the check-ups in some other way since the insurance plan only covers the emergency services and illnesses that suddenly arise. These are services that could have potentially broken the handler's saving bank account. The pet wellness plan is what would be needed to simply cover the routine check-ups.

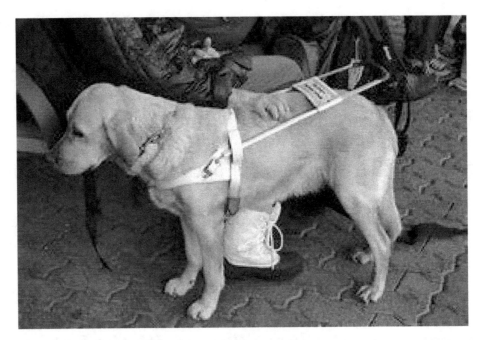

So, what do you get with a pet insurance plan?
With insurance coverage, you get several coverage benefits. Many of these covered services can be quite expensive without an insurance plan and although we all think this will never happen to us, it usually does.

With an insurance plan, you will have coverage for:

- Surgery

- Illness

- Accidents

- Orthopedic conditions

- Emergency care

- Therapy

- Hereditary and congenital conditions

- Prescription medication

- X-rays

- MRI's

- Hospitalization

- Cat Scans

- Ultrasounds, etc.

What do you get with a Wellness Plan?

With a wellness plan, you get coverage for all those things that are not covered by a traditional pet insurance plan. This can include several benefits that will last you for years to come since your dog will need many rounds of shots and check-ups.

The coverage options you will receive when purchasing a pet wellness plan is listed below:

- Teeth Cleanings

- Annual Exams

- Urinalyses

- Spay/neuter

- Flea, tick and heartworm treatments

- Routine vaccinations (rabies, DHLP, Bordetella, Parvo, Lyme, giardia)

- Routine blood panels

- Heartworm testing

- Microchip

- Fecal testing

With pet insurance, oftentimes, you are able to include a wellness plan as an add-on. However, not all insurance plans offer this wellness plan as an add-on. Several of the options that you have for purchasing a pet insurance plan and a wellness add-on plan will be discussed in detail below, so you can see the benefits that each one will offer your Psychiatric Service Dog.

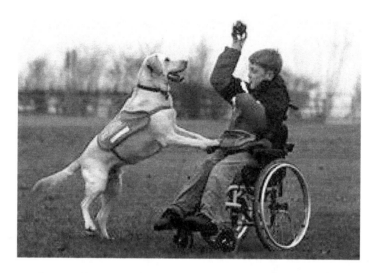

PetsBest Routine Care Coverage with Wellness Plans

Pets Best Routine Care Coverage Plan is one of the most popular options. They have two coverage options for the wellness plan. These are:

- BestWellness

- EssentialWellness

These are additional products that can be added to the insurance plan that you purchase for your pet. Each one covers many different treatments and services. Although they cover these wellness services, there is a per item limit that must be understood. You must also add your wellness package within 30 days of purchasing the pet insurance plan, as well as within 30 days of the insurance plan's renewal. The coverage costs anywhere from $14-30 per month, and this depends on the type of plan you choose to purchase for your pet, as well as whatever state you live in. It also has a rating or cap per item, which means the wellness plan will only cover the vaccinations for $80 and the annual exam at $50. If your veterinarian charges more, you would need to cover the difference.

With this plan, you will have no deductibles for services rendered, and your coverage will begin the day after you pay.

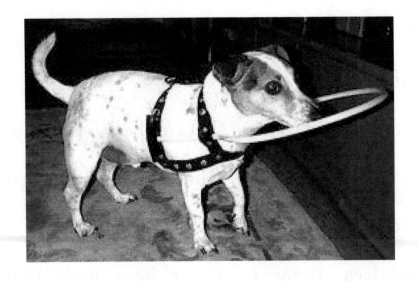

The breakdown for PetsBest can be seen in this friendly little chart.

	EssentialWellness	BestWellness
Per month	$16 for every state but Washington where it is $14	$26 in every state but Washington where it is $30
Spay/neuter- teeth whitening	$0	$150
Rabies	$15	$15
Flea/tick prevention	$50	$65
Heartworm Prevention	$30	$30
Vaccination/titer	$30	$40
Wellness exam	$50	$50
Heartworm test with FELV screen	$25	$30
Blood, Fecal, Parasite Exam	$50	$70
Microchip	$20	$40
Urinalysis or ERD	$15	$25

Deworming	$20	$20
Total Annual Benefits	$305	$535

24PetWatch Wellness Coverage with Wellness Plans and Advanced Wellness Plans

This insurance plan has 2 additional coverage options for a wellness plan. Each one of these plans will have limits to what it covers. These plans start at $10 per month for the routine wellness add-on and the $25 per month advanced wellness coverage. With this plan, there is no deductible. I have included a chart below for you to see the differences in coverage. This will help you see the differences between two diverse types of coverage options between the two companies.

	Routine Wellness	Advanced Wellness
Dental Cleaning Fecal screen	N/A	$100
Heartworm/flea prevention	N/A	$55

Heartworm test or FELV screen	$15	$15
Microchip procedure and or urinalysis	$20	$20
Spay/neuter procedure and or wellness blood test	$80	$100
Wellness exam	$40	$50
Canine Bordetella vaccine/titer or feline FELV vaccine/titer	N/A	$15
Canine DHLPP vaccine/titer or Feline FVRCP vaccine/titer	$15	$15
Rabies vaccine/titer and/or Lyme vaccine/titer, or FIP vaccine/titer	$15	$15

ASPCA Pet Health Insurance with a Preventative Plan

The ASPCA offers 2 separate preventative plans that cover the routine services that are used to keep your Psychiatric Service Dog from getting ill. This is a basic plan that has limited services compared to a prime plan that has more services provided outside of the ones offered by the basic plan. These preventative plans will be covered under the Hartville brand. With the preventative plan, there is no waiting period as well as no deductible.

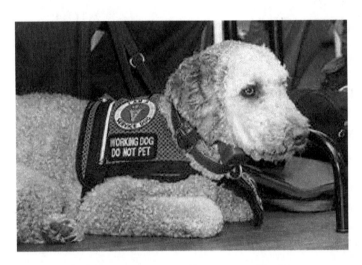

Below is a chart to help you understand the coverages that are available to you through this plan.

	Basic	Prime
Per month	$9.95	$24.95
Dental cleaning	$100	$175
Rabies or Lyme vaccination/titer	$20	$25
Flea/heartworm prevention	$0	$50

DHLP vaccine/titer	$20	$25
Bordetella vaccine/titer	$0	$25
Fecal Test	$20	$25
Wellness exam	$50	$50
Heartworm test	$20	$25
Blood test	$0	$25
Microchip	$20	$40
Urinalysis	$0	$25
Health Certificate	$0	$25
Deworming	$20	$25
Total Annual Benefits	$250	$500

As you can see, each one offers two different purchase options for the wellness add-on with an insurance plan. Each one has a set amount of coverage and provides you with several preventive measures or testing options. With stand-alone insurance, this only covers a few emergency situations and illnesses that arise when they are unexpected.

The benefits that are offered for a wellness plan can include several of these options.

- Wellness exams

- Microchipping

- Grooming

- Deworming

- Parasite prevention

- Vaccinations

- Behavior training

- Dental care

- Spaying/Neutering

- Routine screenings

And when combined with an insurance pet plan, you can gain added benefits that will help in those times of emergency need. These benefits include the ones listed below.

- Accidents

- Orthopedic conditions

- Hereditary and congenital conditions

- Illnesses

- Prescription medications

- Emergency care

When you sign up for a wellness plan, you are able to only pay for what you use, and it is covered by a small monthly payment. With insurance, you will pay a monthly fee that will provide you coverage with an annual limit, a per-incident deductible, and a reimbursement rate with no routine care. This will determine how much your monthly cost will be based on the percentages or limit that you have for services per year.

Below is an example of what you can expect when signing up for the insurance policy for your pet.

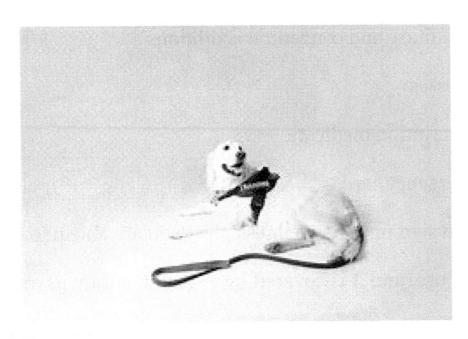

PetFirst Insurance

Annual limit	$10,000
Per incident deductible	$250
Reimbursement rate	80%
Routine care	N/A
Monthly rate	$80.50

Annual limit	$10,000
Per incident deductible	$250
Reimbursement rate	80%
Routine care	$250
Monthly rate	$97.50

PetPlan

Annual limit	$10,000
Per incident deductible	$100
Reimbursement rate	90%
Routine care	N/A, lab tests, dietary supplements, End of life euthanasia,
Monthly rate	$50.72

Embrace

Annual limit	$15,000
Per incident deductible	$750
Reimbursement rate	80%
Routine care	N/A, wellness coverage $250, lab $10,000, dietary supplements $250 as part of the wellness plan, End of life and burial $10,000, $250, end of life euthanasia $10,000, Travel coverage $10,000 injuries and illness only.
Monthly rate	$21.02

Trupanion

Annual limit	unlimited
Per incident deductible	$250 per condition

Reimbursement rate	90%
Routine care	N/A, lab-unlimited, dietary supplements-unlimited, End of life and burial-unlimited, end of life euthanasia-unlimited, Travel coverage-unlimited-injuries and illness only.
Monthly rate	$35.04

ASPCA

Annual limit	$2,500 lifetime annual limit
Per incident deductible	$250
Reimbursement rate	70%
Routine care	$2500-unlimited with additional preventative care, travel coverage without home visit inside the US and Canada
Monthly rate	$12.89

Each one of these companies has a different standard on which they base their coverage, and each one of these rates is being shown with various levels of coverage. This is to give you a basis with which you can apply for coverage. We all have varying needs and income levels, as well as dogs. These rates are based on a younger dog, an Australian Shepherd, with no pre-existing conditions or genetic markers.

As you can see, you are able to opt for an insurance plan that is a stand-alone policy, or you can opt into an insurance plan and wellness package. If you are not concerned about injuries or accidents happening with your dog, then a wellness stand alone is another option that may be the right choice for you. Whatever you choose is based on your needs, your financial abilities, and your availability within your area.

CHAPTER 6: GOVERNMENT REGULATIONS

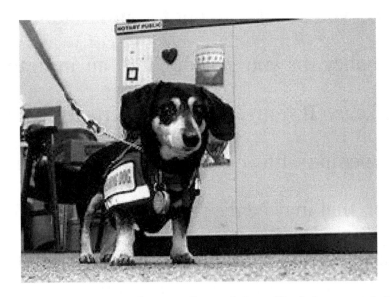

Since the government has a hand in all things within the US, I will go over a few of the regulations that are the deciding factors you need to consider when training your own Psychiatric Service Dog. The Americans with Disabilities Act has specific coverage that pertains to the laws about individuals with disabilities, housing, public access spaces, traveling, and much more. They also help to identify what a person with disabilities or impairment is and how to acknowledge the Psychiatric Service dogs that are cared for by those that are disabled and their rights as disabled individuals. The ADA states that disabled and impaired individuals who have a Psychiatric Service dog will need to have access to their Psychiatric Service dog at all times, and thus are allowed to bring them to the doctors, hospital, on a plane, train, bus or any other public access facility or transport. It also states that housing has to make reasonable accommodations for the person that is disabled to live with their service animal.

How Do I Register My Psychiatric Service Dog?

In order to have a Psychiatric Service Dog, it needs to be trained properly. As per the laws under the ADA, you do not have to pay someone to train your dog for the services that you need. However, it does need to provide an actual service outside of making you feel emotionally better. The diverse types of tasks that your dog can perform for you are based on your Psychiatric needs. The Psychiatric Service dog needs to provide a service for the disabled individual based on their disability. These tasks can include:

- Redirecting or interrupting a compulsive behavior that is destructive.

- Locating something that the disabled person may need or helping them find a safe place when disoriented in a large crowd.

- Searching through a room for someone that struggles with PTSD.

- Providing guidance for the handler who suffers from dissociative disorders.

- Alertness to sounds that can be alarming for the handler or to smoke, as well as security alarms when they sound off.

- Aid with balance for a handler in need of security and walking support.

- Locate and bring medication or other objects to the handler at the times that it is needed.

The next step once your dog is trained for the specific service that you will need is to make the decision on whether or not you want to register the Psychiatric Service Dog for a Psychiatric Service dog registration organization's certificate. Registering is not a necessary step since it is not a legal requirement. The benefit of registering is that they can provide you with an identification card for your dog, as well as vests, ID badges, and a certificate that shows they are a registered Psychiatric Service Dog. These things will be particularly useful when you head out into the world with a Psychiatric Service Dog, especially a vest. Often times, you will be asked if the dog is a Psychiatric Service dog, and sometimes they even ask for proof, although it is very illegal for them to do so. If you decide to go this route, make sure the company you register with is a reputable company. This will ensure that the certification is legitimate.

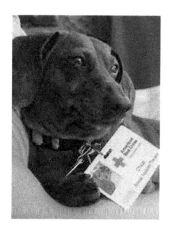

The ADA for Owners of People with Psychiatric Service Dogs Owners

Under the ADA, only dogs are recognized as Psychiatric Service animals. This means that as a Psychiatric Service dog, they are acknowledged under the ADA laws and standards. These standards have been set in place for a number of years. The definition of a Psychiatric Service dog is a dog that is trained to perform a specific task that is useful to the disabled individual's disability. This dog should be able to perform specific tasks as well as perform work that relates to the disabled person. Any public access building or facility must allow the Psychiatric Service dog to accompany the disabled individual in all areas that the public or a member is allowed to go.

Service animals qualify as working animals, not pets, and the tasks must be causally related to the disabled person's disability. If the dog is only providing comfort or emotional support, then they do not qualify as a service animal under the ADA. However, they do fall under the Emotional Support Animals Standard that is set by the Housing Authority. Although this definition for service animal can be limiting, it does not affect the broader definition of assistance animal that is described under the Air Carrier Access Act.

There are several states and local laws that provide a broader definition than the ADA would provide. This information is found through the states' Attorney General Office.

Where can I take my Service Animal?

Due to the laws that are set by the ADA, your local and state government and several nonprofit organizations that provide services for the public have to allow a service animal within their facility to accompany the disabled individual. These accesses only apply to the areas that the public has normal access to. A service animal can enter a hospital with a patient that is disabled, as well as cafeterias, examination rooms, and even ER's. However, if the entry of a service animal would cause issues for the area or people within the area, then the service animal can be excluded. These include operating rooms or burn units since the presence of the service animal could create an unsterile environment.

What can exclude an individual service animal from having access?

The service animal must be under the handler's complete control at all times while in the building. They must be harnessed, leashed or tethered unless the use of these accessories would hinder the service animal's service work for the individual, or the disability prevented the use of these accessories. If this is the case, the disabled person has to have complete control of the animal by voice or signal command.

If the service the dog is performing for the disabled person is not readily obvious to the business owner, then they are allowed to ask a limited amount of questions to ascertain that the dog is a service animal. They may only ask two questions to the disabled person about the service animal.

- Is this service animal required due to a disability?

- What task is the service animal providing for the disabled person?

The staff is not allowed to ask any questions about the disability of the person, nor ask for medical documentation. They cannot require an ID for the dog or any type of training certificate. They cannot ask for the dog to demonstrate its ability to do its task or be shown the task that it performs.

The fear of a dog is not a valid excuse to exclude the service animal from entry. It can also not be excluded from allergies. If there is a person in the same classroom or homeless shelter with someone that has an allergy to dogs or pet dander, then an accommodation has to be made for each person to be comfortable. They must be provided a separate space to sit in or sleep in if there is a possibility for this.

Those with a disability cannot be asked or forced to remove a Psychiatric Service dog from the property of a business or public access facility unless these two things happen.

- The dog becomes out of control, and the handler cannot handle them.

- The dog is not potty trained.

If this takes place, then they have to offer the individual with the service animal the opportunity to purchase the things they need with the presence of the service animal.

If the establishment sells food or prepares food, then they have to provide the service animal the right to enter public areas, even if the local or state health codes prohibit the entry of animals within the area.

A disabled person that is using a service animal cannot be separated from the other people within a facility or business due to the service animal and cannot be charged extra fees for that service animal. If the business requires deposits for guests with pets, this fee must be waived for the service animal.

If a hotel charges guests for damage from themselves or their pets, they are allowed to charge for anything damaged by the guest or the Psychiatric Service dog.

The staff within a hotel or business is not required to provide any services or food to the service animal. Nor are they required to provide care for the service animal.

Although this book is about a Psychiatric Service Dog, there are a few laws that provide Miniature Horses a few rights under the ADA laws. If the Miniature Horse provides a service or performs tasks for a disabled person, they fall within the guidelines of a service animal. This is further defined by what a Miniature Horse would be. They are 24 inches up to 34 inches tall when measured from the bottom of the hoof to the top of the shoulders. They also must weigh between 70-100 pounds. If the disabled person is using a Miniature Horse as a service animal, then they must be provided reasonable accommodations. There are 4 ways to assess the Miniature Horse to determine the accommodation within the facility.

- Is the Miniature Horse potty trained?

- Is the Miniature Horse under the handler's control?

- Does the facility have space to accommodate the Miniature Horse's size, type, weight, and such?

- Will the presence of the Miniature Horse compromise the safety requirements that legitimately provide a safe operational facility?

Housing Authority for Owners of Psychiatric Service Dog Owners

Under the 504 that is outlined in the Rehabilitation Act of 1973 within the Americans with Disabilities Act, they define service animals as animals that aid those that are disabled. However, the Department of Justice limits this definition to only dogs and then excludes emotional support animals from being defined as a service animal. Under the Housing Authorities, emotional support animals are covered for reasonable accommodations as an assistance animal. What this means is that a person with a disability can expect reasonable accommodations when renting a place and having a service animal or emotional support animal. The FHA and the ADA cover housing that is public or ran by a leasing office or real estate office, as well as housing for universities.

Title II law applies to housing that is public entities, as well as government housing and universities. Title III applies to rental offices and shelters, along with multifamily dwellings, facilities that provide assisted living, and public education housing. The 504 also provides covers for those houses that receive financial assistance for their housing needs. HUD covers all types of housing. This will include privately owned and federal assisted houses. However, there are some limited exclusions that are exceptions to the rules. In housing situations where there is a no pets rule, the property owner must allow and provide reasonable accommodations for disabled individuals who have or wish to have a service animal. Since an assistance animal is not a pet, the no pet policy, pet deposit, or pet rent does not apply to these animals. The definition of a service animal has been described throughout this book several times, and it pertains to this definition as well.

For reasonable accommodations, there is no governing law that requires the dog to be individually trained by a specific program or certified or registered under any specific organization. Dogs are the only ones covered as service animals. However, an emotional support animal is an animal that provides emotional support to the individual. If the request is submitted for a resident to use an assistance animal, then they must follow the general principles that are applicable for the accommodations that have been requested. They must then consider these things to assess the accommodation.

- Does this person have a disability?

- Does this disabled person have a service animal that provides a service for their disability? Or emotional support, which helps with the alleviation of the person's disability symptoms?

If the answer is no to either one of these, then the accommodation is not required, and the request could be denied. If the answer to each question is yes, then the accommodation must be made. The only exclusion is if the accommodation would create undue financial burdens or alter the fundamental nature of the said property.

For instance, if the service animal has shown that they are a direct threat to others' safety and cannot be changed by another accommodation, then they can be denied, or in the case where the specific animal in question would cause damage to the property that cannot be eliminated or avoided by another accommodation.

This cannot be based on the size of the dog, the breed, or the weight. And to deny the animal, the decision must be based on that individual animal and not a generalized fear or speculation. Nor can it be based on a previous service animal or dog in the past.

The restrictions or conditions that are applied to pets within housing communities cannot be imposed on a service animal. For instance, the pet deposit does not apply to a service animal or emotional support animal, nor does the monthly rent. Denial cannot take place based on the housing owner's uncertainty about the person's disability or need for a service animal's services. If the disability is not apparent, they can ask for reliable documentation that is provided by a physician, psychiatrist, social worker, or other mental health professionals to explain the need for the service animal. This will provide enough documentation. The letter does not have to be specific about the disabilities of the patient.

They cannot, however, ask for the person to submit medical records or provide them access to the provider of their medical needs. They also cannot request them to provide details as well as extensive material evidence about their disability with documentation from a clinical examination. Each reasonable accommodation request is individually assessed for each person. They cannot conditionally deny the accommodation or charge a fee such as a deposit as terms for the applicant's service animal to be allowed. They also cannot delay the response for an unreasonable amount of time.

If you find that you are denied unfairly, then contact the HLTD to file a complaint about the denial.

Although emotional support animals are covered under the HUD guidelines, they are not considered service animals. They simply provide emotional support, comfort, companionship, and well-being support for the disabled individual. Because of the definition of a service animal, only a dog, as well as a Miniature Horse, can be considered a service animal under the ADA. With this said, I will proceed to the next chapter, where I will start to give in-depth details about how to train your Psychiatric Service Dog for the specific services that you need.

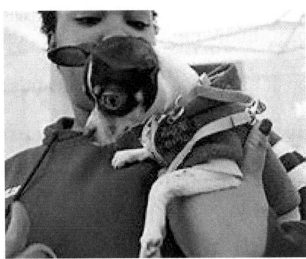

CHAPTER 7: PUBLIC ACCESS REQUIREMENTS FOR A PSYCHIATRIC SERVICE DOG

What they need to know to enter buildings, fly on planes, and such

Public Access Skills

As an owner of a Psychiatric Service dog, you are required to train your dog to perform certain tasks, as well as make sure that they are under control at all times while out in public. There are a few things that you will need to make sure your dog is properly trained before they are allowed to be on public transportation or out in public buildings as a Psychiatric Service dog. These things are listed below.

- Sit on command in various situations - the Psychiatric Service Dog needs to understand that when you say sit, it sits in, and it stays without trying to get up and wander around.

- Controlled loading into and unloading out of a vehicle - they need to be under control while being loaded into a vehicle or unloaded from a vehicle.

- Down on command in various situations - They need to understand and respond appropriately when you tell them to lie down.

- Controlled approach to a building - They need to be completely under your control when they approach a new building or any building for that matter.

- Controlled entry and exit through a doorway - They need to be under control when entering new buildings or existing buildings that they have already visited. Doorways can be scary for a dog, and entering through one is necessary for most activities.

- Control when the leash is dropped - If you happen to drop the leash, they need to be under your control and not chase after animals, people, or simply wander off.

- Control in a restaurant - They need to be able to lie underneath the table at a restaurant and not present a problem for the restaurant.

- Heeling through a building - They need to be able to heel while in a building and not create any problems.

- Six-foot recall on lead - They need to be comfortable on a six-foot recall lead and not try to pull away or cross the path of others.

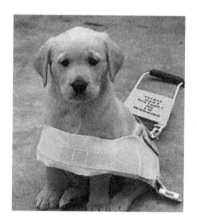

How they need to react with other animals and people

A service animal needs to respond to people and animals as if they are not present. Most service animals wear vests, and these vests will say that they are a service animal and ask for no one to pet them. Although this is recommended for some animals, there are sometimes when I have been able to pet a service animal. It is a good rule of thumb to ask the handler if it is ok before approaching the dog. A dog that is aggressive towards children or other people is not a proper Psychiatric Service dog.

When the Psychiatric Service dog is walking down the street, they should be completely oblivious to the other animals on the street or the other people. It should be hyper-focused on what the handler is doing and if the handler needs any help.

The next two chapters are all about the Psychiatric Service Dog training techniques for specific services that can be performed by the dogs and whom they will benefit. One of the training techniques is on retrieving, and this is something that all people with disabilities can use to help them with their daily life.

CHAPTER 8: STEP BY STEP TRAINING OF A PSYCHIATRIC SERVICE DOG

Every service animal performs a specific task that is taught to them to assist you in your needs in being disabled. Although each service animal needs to have a basic obedience training course prior to being trained for service, they can actually start training for the obedience and then the service that you need them for at the same training course. You do not have to pay a trainer to train your dog for you. In fact, it is better than you train them yourself so that you are both acquainted with the training steps and so that you can have the pack leader established.

For Anxiety and Depression Patients

A Psychiatric Service dog for Anxiety or depression will need to perform certain tasks to qualify as a Psychiatric Service Dog. These tasks can include:

- Providing comfort and support

- Collecting medication

- Using tactic stimulation to divert the handler's attention by licking the face.

- Be able to identify the signs of a panic attack or the onset of a panic attack.

- Provides a sense of purpose and job to the disabled person. Provides a reason to get out of bed or go outside. Feeding, walking and caring for the dog.

A Psychiatric Service dog for depression is a great resource for those that struggle with leaving their homes, especially if that person is in a constant state of depression or negative thoughts, as well as when suicidal. They can help the depressed person live a fuller life.

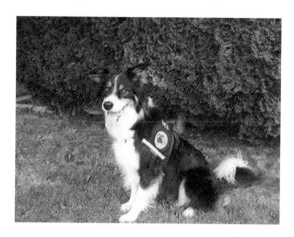

So how do you train your Psychiatric Service Dog for Dep-ression tasks?

First, you must start with the basics. Make sure that your dog has

basic obedience training, such as the type you would find when

signing your dog up for the Good Citizen Training.

All dogs need to have certain basic skills to begin with for

being trained for their Psychiatric Service. Below are the skills

that are
  • Sit and stay
necessary to be trained from the beginning.
  • Down

  • Up

  • Heel

  • Come

- Leave

- As well as potty outside on cue

If you are not equipped to train your dog for these simple tasks, then you will need to find a trainer that can do this for you. You should also consider paying someone to train your dog for the service that you need after the obedience is learned.

Next, you will need to determine what service the dog will be doing for you. As with most disabilities, you will need to have some way of obtaining a phone when you do not have the ability to walk or move. This is a continuing problem for those that have mobility issues as well as the elderly and those that get severely depressed. So, training your dog to retrieve is a great task for them to learn. Another task for anxiety is to identify when an anxiety attack is coming and provide tactile stimulation by licking the person or nudging the handler so that they can begin to pet the dog to reduce the anxiety and calm down quickly.

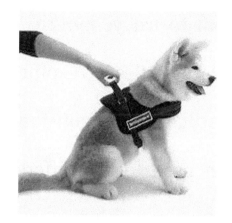

Step-by-step process for training a dog to retrieve:

To do a formal retrieval, the Psychiatric Service Dog would need to be trained to take hold of an object, carry that object, and release the object into the trainer's hand. This process will take patience and determination. You will also need a profound sense of humor to accomplish this. Retrieving allows the dog to pull open doors, pick up an item that is dropped, get the phone, carry some bags, deliver a message to someone, help someone get dressed or undressed, and so much more. If you use your hands, the Psychiatric Service dog will use their mouth. It is vital that you go slow and create a pattern.

Motivational Technique for Retrieval

You can start as young as 5-7 weeks old when teaching this technique.

Start by teaching them to carry, mouth, or play with different textures. Offer them glass bottles, PVC pipe, short pieces of metal, key rings, and toys that have slick, non-fun or cool textures while supervised. If they get used to the different textures, it will be easier to teach them to retrieve objects.

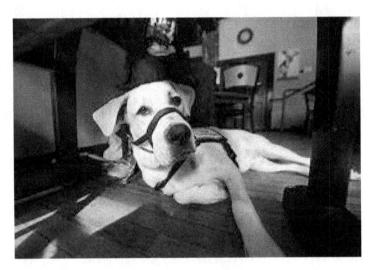

Prior to starting
Understand how to mark behaviors with a clicker. The timing must be impeccable, and you must be confident. This is a process that will take a long time to accomplish.

Condition the pup or adult dog by a clicker in their training

Conditioning the dog to focus on the clicker for a brief period of time, and understanding the basic targeting techniques is a must.

What supplies will you need?

- Dumbbells are useful when teaching them to retrieve something. You can also use a retrieving dummy.

- Clickers

- Treats that have high value or are your dog's favorite treat. This can be things such as chicken bites, hot dogs, or other kinds of treats.

Targeting the Psychiatric Service dog

- Using a chair, sit down and have your Psychiatric Service dog face you.

- Hold out the dumbbell with the clicker.

- Place treats on the other hand.

- Show the dumbbell to your dog. Then click the clicker and place the treat in front of the nose and bump it.

- Move your dumbbell from one side to the other and continue to click the clicker while targeting the nose to bump the dumbbell and then give the dog the treat for the bump.

- Do not pay any attention to your dog's pawing or vocal commands. Only pay attention to nose bumps and then giving it the treat.

- Continue to practice these processes of targeting the dumbbell with the clicker and nose bumping, then giving the dog a treat until the dog focuses and moves a few feet in the direction of the dumbbell and nose bumps it.

Once they have targeted the dumbbell and are doing this process properly, they are ready to start mouthing the dumbbell.

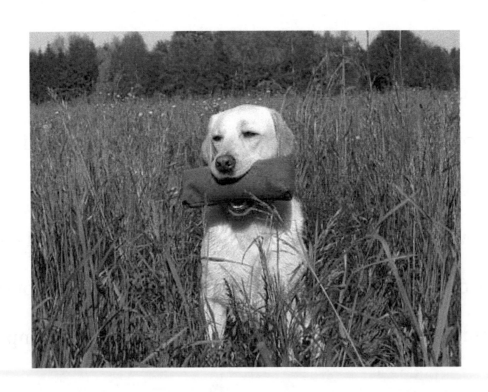

Mouthing the Psychiatric Service Dog

- Start by not clicking for nose bumps and just simply waiting. Do not offer leads or cues to the dog. Once the dog gets frustrated nose bumping the dumbbell without a response, it will open its mouth. Instantly click and give the dog several treats in a row. This is the response we are going for. If the dog does not touch the dumbbell that is ok, simply click, and then provide the treatment for the gaping mouth.

- Continue this process by ignoring the nose bumps but clicking and then providing a treat when the mouth opens. If he happens to brush the dumbbell with his mouth or teeth even if by accident, then click and give him a treat.

- Continue to work on this until the dog purposely opens his mouth and places it on the dumbbell, even if he instantly spits it out. Click the clicker and then give him a treat. This is training the dog to mouth the dumbbell to contact.

- Once the dog has this down, start to only give the dog a treat when he does actual grabs of the dumbbell. This means that the mouth is open, and the teeth close down around it, even if for a split second. Click the clicker and then give the dog a treat.

The next part of training a Psychiatric Service dog to retrieve is teaching distance, duration, and distraction techniques. This helps increase the understanding the dog has of the behavior or command that you are cueing them for. Take each one of these, one step at a time, since they get distracted and can be confusing.

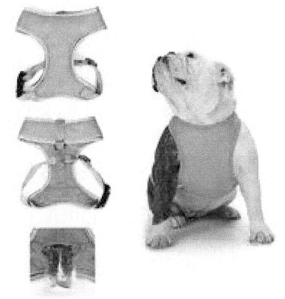

At this time, the Psychiatric Service dog should be looking for a treat as soon as she hears the clicker. She should also grab the dumbbell or retrieving dummy as soon as you present it to her. Do not worry if she immediately spits it out. Your Psychiatric Service dog should also be ok with moving to the left or right a short distance to retrieve the dumbbell.

Introducing your release cue

Although it seems backward to train to release before training to hold, once they learn that they will be releasing the item into your hand, they will be able to understand that they need to wait for the cue to release it.

- Make sure that your dog can do a couple of rounds of clicking and then receiving a treat for grabbing the dumbbell. Once you get to around 3-5 reps that are quickly executed, you can move on to the next step in the process. At this point, the dumbbell should be in your hand the whole time.

- Now, you should introduce the release cue that you will be using. Present the dumbbell to the dog. Once she reaches for it and grabs it, allow her to. Then click the clicker and repeat your command for release. As she releases it to give her a treat. Continue to do this several times until the dog begins to pause, even if for just a second, prior to spitting it out. This means she is listening for the cue.

- Click the clicker for the pause between each grab and again for the release of the dumbbell. Continue to use the release command. As time progresses, you will notice a pause that builds in time. Once she starts to extend her pause, give her multiple treats, especially for lengthy pauses. Remember that the click identifies the behavior you wish to teach. Clicking for pause teaches them to pause. Clicking again for release and saying your release cue is teaching to release. Then give the dog treats for the clicks.

- If you can count to one Mississippi between each pause, then you are ready to move on.

Training the dog to release to your hand

Keep these sessions short. They also need to be positive and upbeat. This is going to be a frustrating session for both the handler and the dog. The goal for this session is to train the dog that they will get a reward, but only if the dumbbell is placed in the handler's hands.

- Start with offering the dumbbell to the dog. When she grabs hold of it, let the dumbbell go, moving your hand underneath her chin. This is so the dog can drop the dumbbell in your hand when it lets it go. Click the clicker and give her a treat when saying your release command. If the dog releases the dumbbell prior to the release word, then move your hand out of the way and let the dumbbell fall to the ground. Do not click your clicker and do not give the dog a treat. Just look at the dog and shrug it off, pick up your dumbbell and offer it to the dog again.

- Continue this process 5-6 times in a row.

- Do this routine over and over again. However, do not say your release word. Instead, you need to wait. If the dog drops the dumbbell again, then shrug and say nothing. Pick it up and offer it to the dog again. This time, use the release word and let the dumbbell fall into your palm. Then give your dog several treats.

- Continue to practice these steps. Every 3rd to 5th time, use the release cue randomly. However, do not use the release cue and allow the dog to spit it out. Shrug off the drop and pick up the dumbbell again and offer it to the dog. Allow the dog to grab and then use the cue to release, and let it drop in your palm. Give a treat when done properly.

- Notice when your Psychiatric Service dog purposefully holds onto the dumbbell for a longer time as if waiting for the release cue. Then use the release cue and allow it to drop properly, and then give several treats for reward.

- Continue to do this until your Psychiatric Service dog has succeeded more times than she has failed. Include the purposeful failures in order to show your dog what is not appropriate and reinforce the behavior for waiting until the release cue.

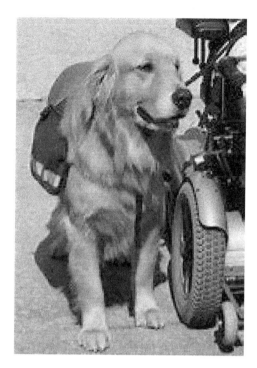

Training for a guided hold

Be very gentle during this phase of training. You are using motivation to train the dog how to retrieve. You do not want to force it.

Have your dog sit beside you. Choose the opposite side of your dominant hand for your dog's position.

- Offer the dumbbell to the dog with your dominant hand. Once her teeth close on it, allow the dog and then slide your hand underneath the dog's chin.

- Stroke upwards on the dog's neck to the tip of her chin with your dominant hand. Do this for a second or two, and then stop. Next, place the dominant hand underneath to catch the dumbbell, clicking to tell the dog to hold. Then using the release cue, allow the dog to release it, and then give the dog a treat.

- Continue this process while increasing the time that the dog holds by 1-2 seconds each time, but only if the dog is calmly holding the dumbbell. If the dog is struggling, trying to spit it out, or moving around, continue to use the soft stroking technique. Take this gentle and slow. Be patient and steady with the hold. It is not a race.

- Continue to do this until the hold reaches 30 seconds with a comfortable or calm hold while stroking the chin gently.

Training the dog to hold

- Start this process as you would the guided hold. Offer the dumbbell to the dog and continue to gently stroke under the chin one to two times. Take your hand away from the chin and after a few seconds, click the clicker. Use the release cue and give the dog a treat. Once the dog releases, pet your dog calmly. If the dog does not wait for the cue to release, then simply shrug it off and pick it back up and try again.

- Repeat this process 2 or 3 more times, and then stop to stroke your dog's chin after she has taken the dumbbell. Hand it to your dog, take your hand away, and wait for 3 to 5 seconds. Use your clicker, and then cue the release. Once the dog releases it, hand her a treat.

- Over time, continue to build gradually. Gain a second or two of hold at a time. Do this until the dog can hold for at least 30 seconds until they receive the cue to release without any guidance from you.

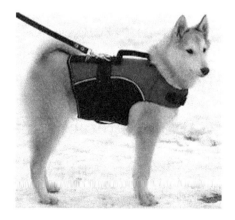

If the dog is continuously failing at this point, then you have too many distractions, or have pushed the dog too fast. Go back to the point at which the dog was succeeding and move forward from that point. Continue to be upbeat about it and set your dog up for a successful training session. If the dog continues to spit out the dumbbell, then continue the shrug and keep quiet. Pick it up and offer it to the dog again. Keep all your sessions short and to the point so the dog will not lose interest and the formal retriever training remains intact.

Train for Desensitizing Touch

At this point, your dog is used to the release cue that you chose. The dog is comfortable dropping the dumbbell into a waiting hand. Remember that this can become an issue for those dogs that start to associate touch with the release command instead of the release cue. If the handler is not ready for the item, then this becomes a problem. To counteract this, you will need to remember that giving the rewards will instill the behavior that you want to train the dog.

- With your dog placed in front of you or on the side of you, begin to desensitize the dog to touch.

- Hand the dumbbell to your dog, remove your hand, and then wait for a few seconds.

- Reach up to gently touch the dumbbell's edge. If the dog drops it, then allow it to fall. Shrug and pick up the dumbbell. Then silently offer the dumbbell again. Reinforce your verbal release cue a few times, and then continue to repeat this light touch again with no cue. If your dog holds the dumbbell, immediately use the clicker and release cue, and then give the dog a reward.

- Hand the dumbbell to the dog and stroke gently on the dog's head or its muzzle. Use the clicker and then give the release command. Once the dog releases, give her a treat for the continued hold and ignore all the drops entirely.

- Continue to work with your dog until the dog waits for the release cue, even if you have curled your fingers around the dumbbell. Stroke your dog's head, muzzle, ears, and touch the dumbbell to show the connection.

Train for Proofing the Hold

Once the dog has happily held the dumbbell for 30 seconds until you cue the release, then you know she has understood the training. This means that your dog understands the take and hold command. Now you need to start proof.

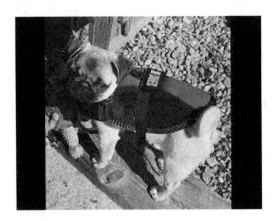

Proofing Game Green Eggs and Ham

This will introduce some variations of the position. Ask for the dog to take and hold while standing or sitting in front of you, as well as position on the opposite side or lying down. Next, have the dog hold it in different circumstances. For instance, standing on the stairs with you a few steps up or down the stairs or in the front seat of your car or in a kennel. Find creative ways to train for a generalized hold behavior. Are the green eggs and ham located in a box? In a car? In a house? With a mouse? Find out what places your dog will continue the take and hold training. Basically, find the wildest and craziest places that the dog will continue the performance standard.

Proofing for Movement and Positions

- Now, you will introduce some movement into the training. Start with asking the dog to change positions while holding the dumbbell. This can start with a shift from side to side or from sitting to standing, a sit to a down, or a stand to a sit, as well as a stand to a down.

- Ask for the dog to make one position change and then reward the dog extensively for the dog's success. Build up 3 or 5 position changes repeatedly, then ask for the release, but take it slow and gradual.

- If the dog starts to drop the dumbbell before you ask for the cue, then you are requiring too much too fast. Go back to a point at which the dog was succeeding, then move forward much slower.

- Once the dog can change its position without dropping the dumbbell, ask the dog to carry it while healing. Start with tiny steps and then build on 30-second intervals for heeling. Reward the dog for success and then ignore her if she drops it. Then, silently pick the dumbbell up and offer it to the dog again.

- Work on a shorter distance instead to increase the dog's confidence level, which in turn, helps the dog succeed.

Proofing the 3 Ds

This is when you will start the 3 Ds. You have started with the duration part of the 3 Ds. The next section is the distance.

- Start with handing the dog the dumbbell, then taking a step back. Pause and then return to your dog. Using the clicker, click and then use the release cue and offer a treat.

- Increase your distance one step at a time until you have acclimated your happy dog to be comfortable with holding the dumbbell and walking 10 steps away, turning, and then coming back to release the dumbbell.

- Once the dog is comfortable with this, increase the distractions that the dog has by adding in the public factor. Try this at a park. Ask the dog to hold the dumbbell while you prepare a meal for the dog or while you are doing basic obedience with a secondary dog.

- Try to be creative with the distractions, but keep your mind focused on the 3 Ds.

- Stay within close range of your dog, and do not expect a long-duration for the hold, especially when introducing the distractions. Be generous with the rewards that you give the dog, and this will ensure the dog's willingness to succeed more than the dog fails. If the dog drops the dumbbell more than the dog holds it, then reduce the distractions that are around the dog and go back to a point where success was better. Gradually increase your difficulty and try again. To reduce the distractibility, move away from the stimulus and slowly move closer to gauge the dog's abilities to perform.

Train Final "Hold" Steps

At this point, your dog is taking, holding, and carrying your dumbbell. This should be a viable action in any situation with your dog. After this, you have smooth sailing ahead.

Continue to proof the hold in all the ways you can dream of. Continue the 3 Ds and continue increasing your distance on walking away from the dog while it is holding. Always reward a job well done. Remember your cue for release, and only click when the release cue is used, and the dumbbell is returned to your hand after a verbalized cue without a simple touch or grab from the handler. Now, you need to combine the carry and distraction training while building on the distance. You are only limited by the creativity that you use to train the dog.

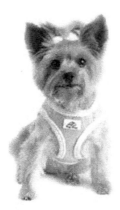

Training To Retrieve a Specific Item or Different Items

To train your dog to retrieve added items, you will need to introduce new objects and start at the beginning. Your dog should notice after about 3-5 items how to retrieve any object that you ask for.

There are several kits that can be used for seeding and add items in the retrieval training process.

- Water bottle

- Glass bottle

- Strips of fleece or cloth

- Metal food bowl

- Spoon

- Spare keys on a ring

- Leash

- Pen

- 12″ section of PCV/Metal Pipe

- Old Credit/ID Card

- Heavy card stock paper

- Large dumbbell

- Key fob

- Empty cans

- Cardboard squares

- Wallet

- Vest

- Small book

- Medicine bottle

- Phone

Train for Things You will Need
Using the seeding kit
You can make your own seeding kit or purchase one. This teaches them odd textures and shapes. Use up to 20 items to train your dog with a seeding kit.

Train for Assisted Pick-Up
- The point is to train the dog to gradually pick up things from a position that is difficult for you to do. So over time, get the dumbbell closer to the ground so that you can train the dog to pick things up from the ground.

- Start in a seated position, then a standing position, bent over position, sitting on the floor, or kneeling over. Whatever you need to do to get the dog to pick up from all positions is simply fine. If at some point your dog stops retrieving on cue, then start again at the last height that where the dog was successful. Then continue to move forward with the steps. Go slow and steady.

- Continue the process that you started with just lowering the dumbbell or item closer to the ground as you continue to train her to take it and hold. Hold the dumbbell as comfortable as you can while holding on. Repeat the process.

- Kneel and continue this process until the dog has this process down for every single level of retrieval. After repeating a couple of times, drop the dumbbell mid-way down your leg, and then repeat the process again.

- Go through this process for each level of retrieval. Continue to train the dog in the take and hold command until you have reached the ground. As you train the dog to retrieve it from the ground, gently remove your hand bit by bit from the dumbbell. This ensures that the dog will retrieve the dumbbell from the ground without your hand on it. Start by using your whole hand, then your palm, then your fingers, then a few fingers, then one finger and so on.

- Lastly, place the dumbbell on the ground and place your hand close to it. Then repeat the steps as before until the dog has the concept down.

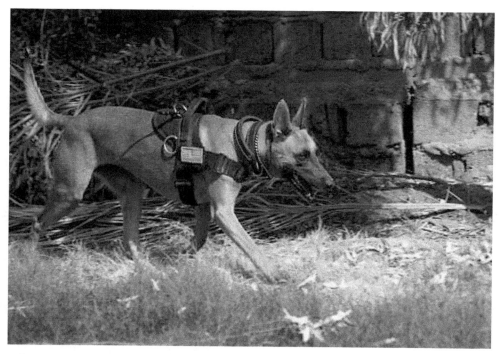

Train for Shaping the Pick-Up

- Instead of holding the dumbbell, place it at a distance from you. Sit in a chair and start the training session with the dog. Instead of speaking to the dog, gaze at the dumbbell every now and then. Once the dog starts to glance at the dumbbell, click the clicker and then offer a treat the moment the dog glances at or lowers its head towards the dumbbell.

- Continue to shape the dog's intuition to pick up the dumbbell by a simple glance. Click the clicker and give a treat for the dog's movements that are appropriate. This can be anything from nudges, nosing, or mouthing the dumbbell.

- Keep quiet and do not use commands or cues to help. The dog should puzzle their way to the correct answer.

- If the dog picks it up, instantly use the clicker to click and give the dog lots of treats. If it picks it up off the ground without assistance, do the same. If it picks it up and then looks at it with a raised head, then repeat the clicker and the reward.

- Repeat this training until you place or toss the dumbbell a distance away from you, and the dog goes to it, picks it up and then waits for the cue to release.

- Repeat these steps while standing, while lying down, or any other position that you may need them to retrieve something for you.

- Once the dog has this down, start using variables and repeat these steps.

Training for Proofing the Retrieve Pick Up

- When standing a distance from the object, ask the dog to retrieve it with the take it cue. If the dog responds properly, then click and reward the dog.

- Repeat this over and over again until the dog performs accurately up to 10 times without any help, do-overs, or hesitations. If this happens, then move on to another object.

- Go back to the Proofing Game Green Eggs and Ham, and train the dog for every item that you will need them to retrieve. Remember the 3 Ds, and be mindful that you only train one at a time.

- This is a formal retrieve from start to finish. Celebrate and reward for this.

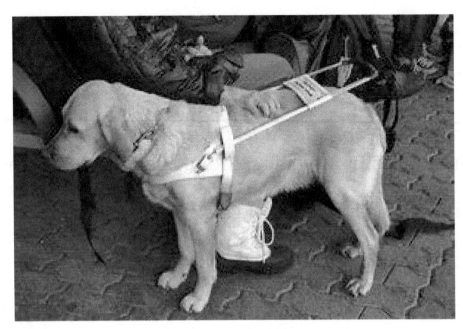

Training for Introducing New Objects

- Start with objects that are similar in shape to the dumbbell and then change it up as the dog learns. Start with the larger items and work your way to the smaller items. Follow these steps to accomplish this about 5 times until the dog picks up the additional items easily. Allow your dog to set their own pace, and if they jump to an immediate pickup, hold and release with cue, then they have the process down.

- Start with a formal retrieval and then add in the added items. Allow the dog to sniff it and explore a bit, making sure to repeat the clicker process with these items. Start from the beginning of the process of the retrieval training for each item. Click and give treats as needed. Build up the hold time and the distance until the dog is retrieving these times on their own.

- Play the Proofing Game Green Eggs and Ham and continue to train the dog.

Train for Retrieval Seeding

Lay two to three items out, with one of them being the dumbbell in a triangle-like pattern. Leave enough space between them for your dog to easily step around them. They still need to be close to each other. Group these items so that the dog does not doubt that they relate. Approach the triangle with the dog beside you and simply say the take cue and point towards the items. Do not specify any item; just allow him to select and pick up the object that he wants. Let the dog hold it, and then use the release command. Give the dog a treat for the actions. Then repeat these steps. Continue to add items to the puzzle until you have introduced all the items to the

Psychiatric Service Dog. Make sure the dog is completely comfortable with these items. Repeat the process until the dog is confident about the puzzle with up to 15 items or more. At this time, start the Proofing Game Green Eggs and Ham and work on your 3 Ds.

Psychiatric Service Dogs for Anxiety

Anxiety is a severe condition that many people suffer from. With a Psychiatric Service Dog, the anxiety sufferer can begin to live a better life. This disorder creates panic attacks, uneasiness, compulsive behaviors and such. You can train your dog to do several tasks for anxiety.

Dogs tend to have close bonds with their handlers and can be trained to identify panic attacks. This would be an individual response style training. I have listed below some steps to take to do this with your Psychiatric Service dog.

Individual Response Training

Start with a dog that has had basic obedience training and then incorporate training steps into training your dog to recognize an anxiety or panic attack.

Start by offering a treat to your dog every time you feel a panic attack coming on. This is a helpful way for the dog to identify the response and know when a panic attack is coming. Another technique to use is cuddling the animal when you feel the stress is coming on. This will help you find relief and help the animal to identify the signs. Finding the right breed is going to be important to train a dog for connecting on this level.

Remember to be patient with the training. Training a dog for public access is important, and this can take up to 120 hours over a 6-month time period. Start with identifying which task the dog will need to provide. They need to identify your heart rate, muscle movements, scratching or touching of your face and other trigger spots, as well as breathing rates. Do you want your dog to lead you away? Do you want them to fetch medication? Do you want the dog to provide safety? Whatever you need to have your dog do, make sure you train for those specific tasks.

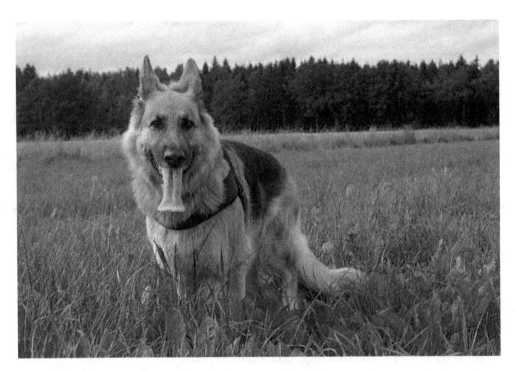

Anxiety alert and detection training
With this training, you will start with the same steps that you did with the previous training. However, you will be teaching them to detect anxiety alerts.

Anxiety cue with treats
- Nudge the dog's nose and reward the dog for the nudge.

- Command the dog to nudge and then add a reward for the dog's actions.

- Repeat this process until the dog has noticed the nudge.

- Change your position in order to train the dog for performing the alert in various locations and seated or standing positions. Reward the dog for each positive response.

- Decide on which anxiety cue to use to help identify the anxiety. This can be the scratching your face or fidgeting as well as rubbing your arms.

- Provide the anxiety cue and act as if the anxiety symptom is real. Then, command the dog to nudge and reward for a positive response.

- Practice this over and over again, the same way you would the retriever process. Start to recognize when your dog identifies the anxiety cue without the command. Reward the identification instead of the command. Ignore any false alerts and shrug them off. Repeat this process several times per day for several weeks.

- As time progresses and the dog learns the trigger, remove the command altogether. Manifest an anxiety episode and leave out the command cue. Reward your dog when they respond appropriately.

- Practice in a variety of various places and positions, and continue to work with your dog until they are identifying regularly.

Anxiety & Reward method for Detect Anxiety

- Identify the anxiety cue you want to use. This can be fidgeting, scratching, or any other active response.

- Use the cue in front of your dog. When the dog recognizes the cue, reward him by giving him a treat.

- Train the dog to nudge you and use a verbal cue for the command.

- Show the dog the anxiety cue and use the verbal command for the alert. When the dog starts to recognize the command and cue, reward it with a treat. When the dog does the nudge while you are experiencing the symptoms, reward your dog.

Ignore any false alerts that the dog may do. Use the same training process and the retrieval training.

- Take the command away and practice using just the physical cues instead of the verbal cues. When the dog alerts to the symptoms for anxiety, then provide the dog with a reward for an appropriate response.

- Add in some complex practice time by adding a variety of circumstances that can be used within different environments with many distractions to train for the anxiety alert.

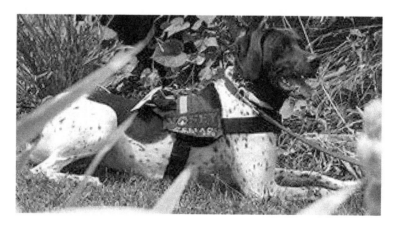

Clicker Training method for Detect Anxiety

- Figure out the alert that you want to use and connect it to the nudge. If the dog nudges your hand, click the clicker and provide the dog with a treat.

- Using a verbal command that is associated with the anxiety, when the dog responds to the command, nudge the hand and then click the clicker when the dog responds properly. Give the dog a treat.

- Manifest some anxiety symptoms and use the verbal cues and physical cues to get the dog's response with a nudge. Then once the dog alerts with a nudge, click the clicker and provide a treat.

- Remove the verbal command and manifest symptoms of anxiety. Next, continue to click the clicker to show the dog that there was a positive response and provide a treat.

- Remove the clicker from the alert command and use the cue for the anxiety symptom to manifest the anxiety. When the dog responds properly, give the dog a reward for responding to the cue.

- Vary your practice in many various places, use distractions and various positions such as sitting, standing, and laying down. Continue to use step 3 if the dog is struggling with this process.

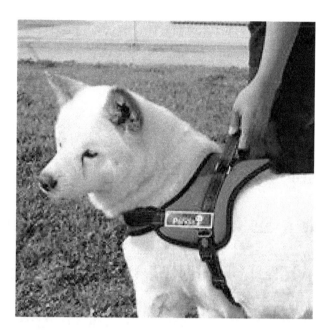

For Someone with Schizophrenia

- Turning on the lights for a person with schizophrenia can be an immense help, especially when they are experiencing an episode. When schizophrenics experience episodes, they can become fearful of the dark because they will see things that are not there, or they will experience voices, and if they do not have lights on, they will think those voices are real.

- Start with standing next to a light switch that you want the dog to reach. Call over your dog and place him in a seated position.

- Hold out a treat on the wall about an inch above the switch. Tap the area a few times and entice the dog to leap up and push the switch with its front paws, right near the switch. If the dog succeeds, then give it a treat and praise.

- Repeat these steps above a few times more until you think the dog has noticed the process of leaping up and touching the wall with its paws. Tap the light switch with your hand while holding the treat on the closed hand. The closed hand should be placed above the switch. Use the command that you chose for turning on/off the light. When the dog's paw has touched the light switch, give it a treat and praise. This is a transition to get the dog used to touch the light for the treat.

- Once you can get the dog to consistently touch the light when you place your hand there, you will be able to place your hand on your side and still get the dog to touch the light. Start with tapping the switch and then rewarding the action when the dog is done and sitting back down.

- Next, you will need to gradually move away from the light switch and use a command or motion to get the dog to use the action of getting the lights for you.

- This can only be used for dogs that have medium to moderate-sized build and ones that are comfortable when balancing on their hind legs. However, some of the smaller dogs are eager to jump up and turn the lights off or on. You may want to purchase a staircase for the smaller breed dogs, though, since they could hurt themselves by jumping

high. Schizophrenics have episodes where they see things or hear things that are not there. Here is a technique to train the dog to help with these episodes.

Dissociative disorder cue with treats

- Nudge the dog's nose and reward the dog for the nudge.

- Command the dog to nudge and then add a reward for the dog's actions.

- Repeat this process until the dog has noticed the nudge.

- Change your position in order to train the dog for performing the alert in various locations and seated or standing positions. Reward for each positive response.

- Decide on which anxiety cue to use to help identify the Dissociative disorder. This can be scratching your face or fidgeting, as well as rubbing your arms.

- Provide the Dissociative disorder cue and Act as if the Dissociative disorder symptom is real. Then command the dog to nudge and reward for a positive response.

- Practice this over and over again the same way you would the retriever process. Then start to recognize when your dog identifies the Dissociative disorder cue without the command. Reward the identification instead of the command. Ignore any false alerts and shrug them off. Repeat this process several times per day for several weeks.

- As time progresses and the dog learns the trigger, remove the command altogether. Manifest a Dissociative disorder episode and leave out the command cue. Reward your dog when they respond appropriately.

- Practice in a variety of various places and positions, and continue to work with your dog until they are identifying regularly.

Dissociative disorder is when a schizophrenic disassociates from the world around them and starts to see and hear things that do not exist. This can also allow them to manifest multiple personalities as well as have moments in their life where they are talking to other people that no one else's sees. These episodes can cause them to see aliens, bugs, people, dogs, monsters and also hear sounds that others cannot. In those moments, they can become violent, rage, aggressive, and even have been known to murder their families and even their own children. Many times, this condition needs to be hospitalized.

In the next chapter, I will continue to discuss the training techniques that can be used to train a Psychiatric Service Dog for various tasks. In this chapter, I discussed anxiety, depression, and schizophrenia. In the next chapter, I will discuss Autism, ODD, IED, and also PTSD.

Each one of the techniques that are discussed in the last two chapters can actually be incorporated for each one of these conditions. It just depends on what you need from your Psychiatric Service Dog.

CHAPTER 9: STEP BY STEP TRAINING OF A PSYCHIATRIC SERVICE DOG CONTINUED

For Autism/ODD/IED

Autism is a world in which the person afflicted with it will live, and it is virtually impenetrable. Those who suffer from Autism have no idea how to connect with emotions or read social cues. They have obsessive behaviors, and it can place a strain on their family. They tend to participate in ritualistic-like behaviors that can be repetitive. This can sometimes last for hours. They tend to flap their arms, spin coins, line cars up, or filter things through their fingers. On the opposite end, they may not like to be touched or require overstimulation with touch. They tend to have higher levels of sensory receptors, and these can cause overloads. They get overwhelmed and have meltdowns without a way to tell you about the problem. This can be difficult to know how to respond. However, a Psychiatric

Service dog can usually help them calm down and prevent more damage when they are raging since they do not have a lot of verbal communication levels. Even the ones that can communicate still do not have the capacity to explain their emotions or what is wrong in those overwhelming moments. Loud noises, as well as lights, can be overwhelming to an autistic child, which may cause a meltdown.

Behavior Intervention

There are several ways to help with autism, and behavior intervention is one of them. One way to provide a behavior intervention is to use a technique for interrupting repetitive behaviors.

Interrupting Repetitive Behaviors

By training a dog to apply pressure on the child's arm for a brief section, you can help interrupt the behaviors. The Psychiatric Service Dog can be trained for specifically stopping these behaviors. They can use a voice command or a physical sign for a cue. Training the dog by action is pretty simple. Earlier, we discussed training a dog to retrieve items and then we discussed using anxiety cues to alert a dog to anxiety attacks. This is no different. In this situation, you can use a trigger such as the flapping and jumping of the child to trigger the dog to place a paw on the child. This works the same way it did prior.

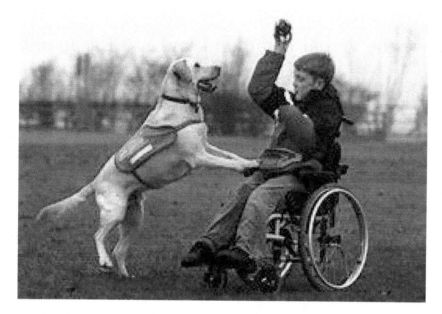

Clicker training method for interrupting behaviors in Autism patients

- Using the alert of jumping and flapping, connect it to the dog's nudge. If the dog nudges your hand, click the clicker and provide the dog with a treat.

- Using a verbal command that is associated with the jumping and flapping, allow the dog to respond to the command, and then nudge the hand. Next, click the clicker when the dog responds properly. Give the dog a treat.

- Manifest some jumping and flapping symptoms with the autistic child and use the verbal command cues to get the dog to respond with a nudge. Then, once the dog alerts with a nudge, click the clicker and provide a treat.

- Remove the verbal command and use the manifested jump and flap symptom so that the dog will identify the trigger. Next, continue to click the clicker in order to show the dog that there was a positive response, and then provide a treat.

- Remove the clicker from the alert command and use the cue for the jump and flap autism trigger to manifest the episode. When the dog responds properly, give the dog a reward for responding to the cue.

- Vary your practice in many various places, use distractions and various positions such as sitting, standing, and laying down. Continue to use step 3 if the dog is struggling with this process.

This can be modified to be used for many different triggers, such as a repetitive word that is used by the patient or hitting their head repeatably. Either way, using the modification for behaviors in this technique will work amazingly. Since Psychiatric Service Dogs are trained very extensively, people often think that the dog is able to judge all situations. However, they are not able to be analytical and use reasoning. So, expecting them to protect your child from a dangerous situation is something that needs to be taught to them. Since the bond between a child and dog is strong, they will notice cues that will help keep the child pretty safe and redirect them in a positive way to another behavior.

Calming and Preventing Meltdowns

Another task that a Psychiatric Service Dog can do for an autistic

child is helping them calm down or preventing a meltdown. They can be trained to aid with meltdowns by applying pressure. In these situations, the dog can be asked to provide deep pressure by being trained to lay on top of the child in a comforting way. In the event that the child is crying, the dog would be able to recognize the sound and snuggle the child to help soothe and calm the child down. Oftentimes, the Psychiatric Service Dog will prevent or reduce the length of the meltdown. This can be done by applying the same steps as above except changing the trigger and response to a different one.

Below is a break down of how this will work. Remember, when training your Psychiatric Service Dog that conditioning is the method with which you are able to train them. If they feel they are getting a positive result, they will be more than happy to help you with the services that you are teaching them. Dogs need positive reinforcement and thrive on a reward system. They will learn easier and be more willing to help you, especially since they are people pleasers.

Clicker Training method for detecting a crying child
- Identify that the child is crying and connect it to the nudge.

  If the dog nudges your hand, click the clicker and give the dog a treat.

- Using a verbal command that is associated with a crying child, teach the dog to respond to the command by nudging the hand and click the clicker when the dog responds properly. Give the dog a treat.

- Manifest some situation of the crying child and use the verbal cue along with the physical cue to get the dog to respond with a nudge. Then, once the dog alerts with a nudge, click the clicker and provide a treat.

- Remove the verbal command and manifest symptoms of the child crying. Once the dog nudges the child, continue to click the clicker and provide a treat. This shows the dog that there was a positive response.

- Remove the clicker and use the cue for the crying child to alert the dog to the child. When the dog responds properly, give the dog a reward for responding to the cue.

- Vary your practice in many various places. Use distractions and various positions such as sitting, standing, and lying down. Continue to use step 3 if the dog is struggling with this process.

- Once the dog has responded continuously with the same process, change the nudge to a deep pressure application and continue to train the dog for this service.

This task will fit the needs as defined by the Service Animal Law and would be allowed in a public building. This would provide extended amounts of service from the dog while the child is in overwhelming situations.

Training a dog to find you

Play hide and seek with your dog. This is the easiest way for your dog to learn how to find you. For instance, if you have an autistic child, and you want the dog to be able to locate the child, train it to find the child. Children that are autistic tend to walk away often. You can quickly help your child to be found when they get lost if you have trained the dog to locate them

- To do this, hide the child behind a tree or wall and ask the dog to locate them.

- Do not allow them to make noises since the dog needs to learn to identify by their smell.

- Once the dog notices the child has disappeared, the dog will start looking for the child on its own. Some dogs may need more time than others to recognize that the child is gone, and others may first get anxious before looking for the child, especially if the child and the dog have bonded.

- This will trigger the dog's natural need to find the child.

- Once the dog starts looking for the child, you can have them make some small noises that will help the dog search. Since no one is completely quiet when they are out in the woods or lost in the home or neighborhood, it will help locate the child quicker.

- Once the dog finds the child, praise the dog for an excellent job and give it a treat.

- By using this method, you are training the dog that it is their job to locate the child when they wander away. Children tend to get lost often due to their natural curiosity. However, autistic children will wander away due to overstimulation or even just the fact that they are prone to bolting.

If you train them with a leash for this task, then the leash is helping with the training situation by speeding things up because your dog will notice that the child is gone by the reduced pressure on the leash.

Using a fenced in backyard can provide a safer area to work in, while keeping the dog in an area that is confined. This will also help with the child that is prone to wandering off. This is effective for both the child and the dog if they are not trained to stay with you. Training your dog to pay close attention to you is part of the basic obedience training that you would have already provided your dog.

If your dog is having trouble finding the child in the beginning, then use a few sounds or noises to call their attention to the child and excite them in a way to encourage them to look for the child. Once they find the child, praise the dog for doing an excellent job. Making the lessons exciting and fun helps keep a slower dog more interested in learning faster and getting good at finding the child.

After playing this game of hide and seek a couple of times a day, the dog should get the idea. At this time, you can then be quiet and give the dog a chance to realize you have not made any sounds to call the dog to you. This will entice them to start wandering around and looking for you. They will be interested in knowing what you are doing and where you are. Be sure to praise them with some treats or petting, and always say "good boy." Encourage them with play and allow them the time to learn to look for the child so they can develop a sense of connectivity to the child and finding it in times of need.

Playing at home is another way to do this task. Anytime the child wants to play with the dog, they can hide inside the house. This will make the dog look for the child. If the child makes noises, the dog will become alert and stand at attention. Then, they will go look for the child and when they find the child. The child can give them a treat. This makes it a game for both the child and the dog. Continue to praise the dog each time it locates the child. After a while, you can stop using noises to get the dog's attention and instead wait for the dog to recognize and start looking.

You can also do this in another fun way by allowing the child to run away from the dog, and all of a sudden, creating a concern for the dog. By calling the child as if the child is gone, the dog will start to look for the child. This will make them look for the child much quicker. Even though you make it seem like a game, they will feel a need to look. By making it a game, the dog is learning, and the child is not in danger. If you like, you can throw one of the dog toys for the dog to go after and then have the child hide while the dog is looking for the toy. The dog will go to collect the toy and come back looking for the child. This will prompt the dog to go look for the child.

You can also use a course for tracking to make the child disappear. AKC dogs tend to be tested on this for titles in tracking. This is often a learned skill that is taught to dogs that track their handlers first or it can be used as a practice for learning how to follow an obstacle course.

You must make the trail or course yourself so that the dog smells your scent on the course. Then the child can travel the trail leaving a scent of them behind. This helps them make a map of the course for the dog to travel down looking for the child.

You can also use clothing to track the scent of an autistic child so that if it gets lost, the dog can find it. One way to do this is to let the dog see the kid wander off but use a shirt to give the dog the scent and let the dog track the child. This should be done with a freshly worn shirt, and that is only touched by the child recently.

By leading the child on the obstacle course, you can drop pieces of clothing of that child so that the dog can track the child through smell. Walk slowly straight ahead in a line for 30 paces and then place another article of clothing that the dog will be able to sniff out and provide treats to reward your dog. Use the child's shoes to scruff the path as the child walks for 20 or 30 paces again, and then leave another scented item such as a toy or shirt. Make sure to give the dog treats as it continues to track.

By allowing your dog to learn to track your autistic child, you are also teaching the dog how to steer the child away from wandering off. Since autistic children tend to wander often, this can be a big deal to parents and can very overwhelming to the child as well when they find themselves lost in strange places.

Leading your dog from a starting point with clothes that smell like the child will help them to identify the child's whereabouts and gain the advantage for the next time they disappear. This is not only for children though. Several adults have severe autism that will cause them to walk off in the same manner. By making it a pattern to hunt the autistic individual, the dog will continuously look out for that individual and make sure that if they do not see them, they start to hunt them down to protect them.

Always encourage the Psychiatric Service Dog to continue forward with the search by allowing it to start the walk in the same direction where the next scented item is located. This allows you to simply tell your dog to find it, and they will head in the right direction from the beginning. It will go and find the trail of scented clothes easily and without trouble. Then, you should continue giving praise and treats, and this will encourage them to continue to look for the child. Over time, the dog will do it like it is second nature, and you can eliminate the reinforcements that are needed to get the dog excited about doing it.

After you have done this a few more times, you will be able to point the dog in the right direction without having to worry too much if the dog will find the child or not since the child's clothing is scented, and your dog will automatically follow the scent of the child or adult that is missing. Leaving a trail for every scented item of clothing helps to connect the dog's nose to the person they need to track and helps them locate places that you have been. This is exactly how the police train their dogs to locate prisoners that have run away.

Obsessive Compulsive Disorder behaviors cue with treats

- Nudge the dog's nose and reward the dog for the nudge.

- Command the dog to nudge and then add a reward for the dog's actions.

- Repeat this process until the dog has noticed the nudge.

- Change your position in order to train the dog for performing the alert in various locations and seated or standing positions. Reward the dog for each positive response.

- Decide on which Obsessive-Compulsive Disorder behaviors cue to use to help identify the Obsessive-Compulsive Disorder Behaviors. This can be scratching of your face or fidgeting, as well as rubbing your arms.

- Provide the anxiety cue and act as if the Obsessive-Compulsive Disorder Behavior symptom is real. Then, command the dog to nudge and reward for a positive response.

- Practice this over and over again the same way you would the retriever process. Then, start to recognize when your dog identifies the Obsessive-compulsive Disorder Behaviors cue without the command. Reward the identification instead of the command. Ignore any false alerts and shrug them off. Repeat this process several times per day for several weeks.

- As time progresses and the dog learns the trigger, remove the command altogether. Manifest an Obsessive-compulsive Disorder Behavior episode and leave out the command cue. Reward your dog when they respond appropriately.

- Practice in a variety of places and positions, and continue to work with your dog until they are identifying regularly.

For PTSD

Training for Psychiatric Service Dog can be broken down into 13

effortless steps when applying deep pressure for a person that

suffers from PTSD. PTSD is a debilitating disorder that prevents

the sufferer from experiencing life and all that it has to offer.

PTSD manifests in many different ways and can come from many

different situations in life. Oftentimes, PTSD can come from the

trauma that is experienced during war or experiences in life,

such

as car accidents, sexual assault, abuse, and many other things.

PTSD patients have several unique needs that can be met by a Psychiatric Service Dog. These can include:

- Help block person in crowded areas

- Interrupting destructive behaviors

- Calm the handler using deep pressure therapy

- Provide security enhancement tasks (such as room search)

- Retrieve medications

- Deep pressure

These 13 effortless steps can mean the difference between living happily and suffering in fear every day while being stuck in your home.

Deep Pressure technique

- Provide some delicious treats for your dog. Sit on the couch and begin to train your dog for the service that you need. By putting a treat in front of the dog's nose, you can slowly move the treat to the back of the couch. Once there, pat the couch back and repeat your dog's name with excitement.

- Once the dog places its front paws on the couch, say "Up! Good!" and then reward the dog with its favorite treat.

- If the dog is a medium-sized dog, you will need to have all four paws on the couch prior to repeating the command "up". Once they are on the couch, train them to lie down.

- If the dog does not place there paws up at first, then you will need to work in stages and reward actions that bring the dog closer to the end result. For instance, when the dog places their head on the couch, place one paw on the couch, then eventually place all paw on the couch. Each time, keep on giving a treat to the dog until you get the result you need. This gets the dog to do a bit more each time. Eventually, the dog will have all the paws on the couch.

- Continue to practice this action until the "up" command gets the result you are looking for. Then, continue until the dog does it without coaxing.

- Once the dog is up, use the command "Okay, Good!" get the dog off the couch. Then proceed to praise the dog. If you use this every time the dog is told to get off the couch, they will learn it from repetition.

- Next, lay down on the couch and use your hand and pat your lap or chest to call the dog up on you. Say, "up!" At this time, the dog may be surprised or worried about climbing on you. It is a normal reaction. Give them a treat for anything that is a positive step towards the end result. Once they relax and understand, they will be less likely to stiffen up. You will have to lure them into this action since they will not be used to this.

- A small to a medium dog can lie on the chest in a spoon or cuddling position with their head next to yours.

- Once the dog has the hang of getting on top of your chest, practice the down command and get the dog accustomed to helping you with deep pressure.

- Do not get frustrated with the dog. They are as new to this as you. If you find that you are frustrated, then stop and take a break. The key is to make this fun and not at all stressful.

- If you have to take a break, then start again later. Sometimes, the dog will get overwhelmed and needs time to recover. This training can take some time for them to adjust to.

- A large dog can apply deep pressure by putting his paws on either hip and lying across your lap or over your breast area.

- Each time your dog gets it right, extend the amount of time they lay there before giving the down command. Use treats and enforce the joy of the task. Eventually, you will be able to eliminate the treats and replace it with praises for a job well done.

If you are using a large dog, then you should teach them to push their head into your torso. Once they get used to the process, they will naturally cuddle you with their head moving closer to your torso. Praise them for this and give them a treat.

If the dog stands on his hind legs, then allow it time to rest its legs before you continue practicing. If you do have a full panic attack this time, rest may not be allowed, but that is ok, the dog will get used to this eventually.

This technique can work with many different psychiatric conditions. Autistic, Depressed, Anxious, PTSD, and other patients can all benefit from this technique.

This book has given you several ways to train a dog for different services that will aid a disabled person with psychiatric needs. Dogs can be a terrific addition to your medical maintenance plan, and they can help give a person back their life. When someone is diagnosed with mental health issues, it can be even more devastating than having the illness. Imagine if you went from working full time to being confined to your home due to fear and panic attacks. Or what if you are moving along in life and then something traumatic happens, and now you are suffering from PTSD.

How would you come to the realization that you may never work again or even get to experience the world like you are used to? This can be an excessively big blow to someone's ego and their social life. But with a Psychiatric Service Dog, you can start to take back the control that you have lost by this illness. Many people are suffering from some form of mental health and even more suffer from autoimmune disorders as well as medical problems such as diabetes. With the specialized training that can be provided to a dog for them to provide therapeutic service to the disabled, there is no limit to what people with illness can do now. You may not be able to work anymore, but at least you can try to experience a world without worry.

Post Traumatic Stress disorder cue with treats

- Nudge the dog's nose and reward the dog for the nudge.
- Command the dog to nudge and then add a reward for the dog's actions.
- Repeat this process until the dog has noticed the nudge.

- Change your position in order to train the dog for performing the alert in various locations and seated or standing positions. Reward the dog for each positive response.

- Decide on which anxiety cue to use to help identify the Post Traumatic Stress Disorder. This can be scratching your face or fidgeting, as well as rubbing your arms.

- Provide the Post Traumatic Stress Disorder cue and act as if the Post Traumatic Stress Disorder symptom is real. Then command the dog to nudge and reward for a positive response.

- Practice this over and over again the same way you would the retriever process. Start to recognize when your dog identifies the Post Traumatic Stress Disorder cue without the command. Reward the identification instead of the command. Ignore any false alerts and shrug them off. Repeat this process several times per day for several weeks.

- As time progresses and the dog learns the trigger, remove the command altogether. Manifest a Post Traumatic Stress

Disorder episode and leave out the command cue. Reward your dog when they respond appropriately.

- Practice in a variety of various places and positions, and continue to work with your dog until they are identifying regularly.

CONCLUSION

Thank you for making it through to the end of *Training Your Own Psychiatric Service Dog*. I hope it was informative and provided you with all of the necessary tools you need to achieve your goals, whatever they may be. Psychiatric Service dogs have been around for a while. And in the past 10 or so years, psychiatric patients have been training their dogs to provide the services as well. It used to be that you had to be blind or deaf to get a Psychiatric Service dog, but those days have passed. I hope this book provided you with the necessary information to help you train your dog and improve your life.

The next step is to start to figure out what exactly your Psychiatric Service Dog will be doing for you and start to look for the perfect Psychiatric Service Dog breed for your needs. Many people are not aware of the regulations that are associated with Psychiatric Service Dogs. Because of this, I have touched on that information within this book. I know that in order for you to be well prepared, you have to know what you are dealing with.

Few people know that they can train their own Psychiatric Service Dog and many people are getting ripped off. This book will hopefully put a stop to that. I hope that you learned how to figure out what the Psychiatric Service Dog breed you would like and also how to train the Psychiatric Service Dog at home for your specific needs.

Finally, if you found this book useful in any way, a review on Amazon is always appreciated!

Printed in the USA
CPSIA information can be obtained
at www.ICGtesting.com
CBHW061747211024
16187CB00042B/1681

DAVID MUEN[CH]

Timeless Moments

Grand Canyon National Park

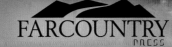

FARCOUNTRY PRESS

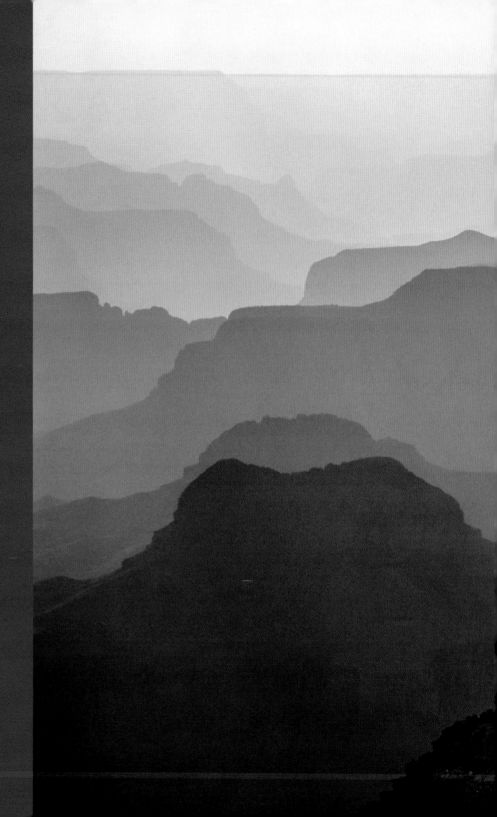

Right: I captured this "timeless moment" just before dark descended from Desert View Point on the South Rim of Grand Canyon National Park. The canyon's backlit ridges show endless gradation of soft evening light.

Title page: On a moody mid-morning in winter, clouds drift across my view from the South Rim of the Grand Canyon to the North Rim.

Front cover: As a winter storm briefly clears, afternoon sunlight brings light and shadow to the iconic formations viewed from near Yavapai Point on the South Rim. The rims below my feet are testimony to the carving power of the mighty Colorado River just barely visible in the depths of the canyon.

Back cover: Looking upstream from Toroweap Overlook, at the far west boundary of Grand Canyon National Park on the North Rim, the Colorado River in shadow and the rock at sunrise captured my imagination. This location was one of my first destinations in the park when I began photographing "timeless moments" in the landscape.

ISBN: 978-1-56037-680-4

© 2017 by Farcountry Press
Photography © 2017 by David Muench

For more information about our books, write Farcountry Press, P.O. Box 5630, Helena, MT 59604; call (800) 821-3874; or visit www.farcountrypress.com.

Produced in the United States of America.
Printed in China.

21 20 19 18 17   1 2 3 4 5

Table of Contents

Foreword by Jeff Kida

My experience with David Muench's photography dates back to 1978, when I first began working in the photography department at *Arizona Highways*. In those days, contributing photographers would send in packets of their recent work from their travels around the state, and the images I most looked forward to reviewing belonged to David. Sifting through his 4x5 transparencies on a light table, I was never disappointed. Each frame included something that differentiated his work from that of other photographers. Sometimes it was his ability to find a new vantage point from an overworked location. Or it might be his lens selection: When everyone was shooting with wide-angle lenses in Monument Valley, David was using a telephoto lens, compressing the iconic buttes against distant mesas. Early on, I realized David had the ability to pre-visualize a scene—to see images in his head before he entered the field. This set him apart as an artist, and it also transported anyone viewing his images, allowing the viewer to become part of his narrative.

David's work was first published in *Arizona Highways* in 1955, and I'm guessing he was on cloud nine when the eighteen-year-old discovered his photo of saguaro cactus was featured on the cover of the January magazine. From that point, David picked up momentum with his work—gracing the magazine pages with greater frequency. His first Grand Canyon images appeared in our June 1960 issue. In particular, one full-page photo made from Toroweap Overlook showed hints of the compositional magic that he would build on for the rest of his career.

From what I can tell, he's never tried to compete with other photographers. He has set his own course, and worked alone. He would study places to see what they had to offer, then set out to capture each site in his own way. Because David set his internal bar so high, he would scout a new location, shoot it, and return year after year to improve on the images from his original take. I have met few people who have the drive to produce his level of work.

Not only is David a student of shadow and light, he's also a student of seasons and weather systems. He would religiously map out trips to Arizona during the summer monsoon season, taking advantage of the massive cloud buildup and the ensuing thunderstorms. Photographers like David look forward to the seasonal shift when what appears pedestrian one morning can become extraordinary in a matter of hours.

Although he's made his own way and worked alone for much of his professional life, David appreciates and honors the work of a number of photographers who preceded him: his father, Josef Muench; Ernst Hass; Edward and Brett Weston; and especially, Ansel Adams. Adams, it turns out, put David's name on a short list for inclusion in the archives of the Center for Creative Photography—high praise from a visionary of landscape photography and one of the founders of the Tucson-based center.

One of the most enduring aspects of David's legacy is his influence on other photographers. His style is emulated by people who don't even know his name. Consciously or unconsciously, photographers adopt certain ways of seeing and a style of shooting, and they have David to thank for it. It's almost impossible to imagine any landscape photographer working today who has not been influenced by David Muench's images. ❖

Facing page: Evening light in the Grand Canyon can create startling reds and purples on the rock layers. As the full moon rose over Wotans Throne and Vishnu Temple, I made this image from Yaki Point on the South Rim.

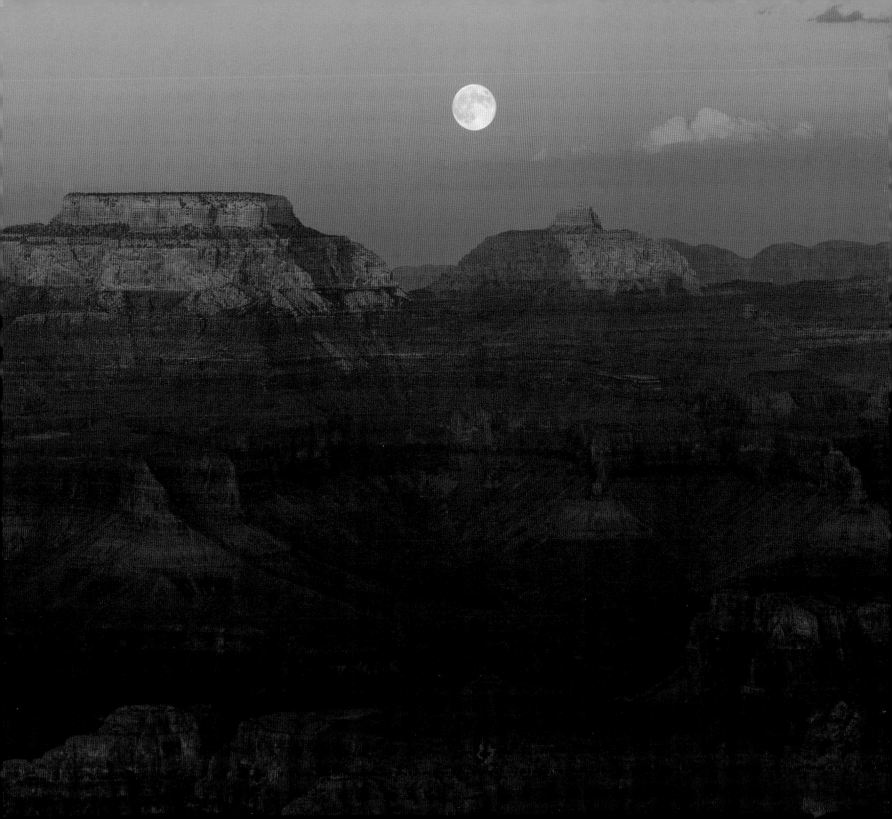

Impressions of the Grand Canyon

I look across the Grand Canyon and the sheer power of nature humbles me. The ribbon of river far below, the force that carved this incredible landscape, created the ultimate chasm in our world. Here I look down from the rim into the interior of geologic time.

Approaching the South Rim, I feel anticipation for that moment I will stand at its edge, seeing and feeling the earth fall away. The silence of time lies out before me. These moments are as exciting as the first rapid on a river trip—the sound, the spray, the inevitable drop—when I am in the canyon's rushing heart. What will I see, on this visit, as the light changes? Will a dramatic storm blow in to reveal a very different canyon than I expected? Will I be able to capture with my camera a timeless moment in this timeless place? This vast, fascinating landscape has drawn me as an artist and lover of this country to return to the Grand Canyon many times over seven decades. Even though I have traveled all over the globe photographing spectacular places, I still feel the Grand Canyon is one of the wonders of the world.

The Grand Canyon itself is the star performer in this collection of photographs made throughout my life. Some of these classic images have been published repeatedly in books, magazines, and exhibits. Others, from my private collection, represent my own personal vision and appear for the first time in this book. My many canyon hikes, river trips, nights spent camping, and dawn location setups to produce hundreds of images just begin to hint at the Grand Canyon's living, unfolding story. I still have much to learn here.

I was a small boy when I first saw the Grand Canyon with my parents. They were passionate nature lovers. My mother, Joyce, a botanist, and my father, Josef, a nature photographer, took me with them on countless road trips. My childhood summers were spent hiking up to viewpoints and down into canyons, watching sunrises and sunsets, running rivers, spending long days with colorful people who hosted us in canyons, valleys, and mountains in the 1950s and '60s. I made my first hike to the bottom of the canyon with my father when I was ten. We stayed at Phantom Ranch one night and in the shelter downstream the next night before hiking back up the South Kaibab Trail. I remember it was very, very hot in the depths of the canyon—and I felt sick from drinking cold lemonade. We made it up to the cooler air at the South Rim that day, although considerably slower than my father's usual fast pace. I have never forgotten that first adventure down to the Colorado River.

Right: My father photographed me enjoying dinner with friends on a river trip through Glen Canyon in the early 1950s. I'm standing at the left. Art Green and my mother, Joyce Muench, are seated in the center with our guides Irene and Earl Johnson (seated right) and their son (kneeling, at left). PHOTO BY JOSEF MUENCH

Facing page: My mother and I often modeled for my father's magazine images, helping "show scale" in the expansive landscape of the West. He made this image of us from below North Rim Lodge in the late 1940s. PHOTO BY JOSEF MUENCH

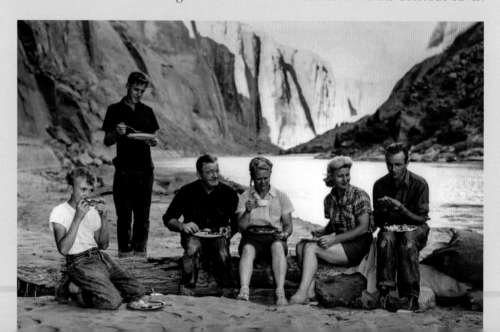

Photography trips with my parents were a big part of my childhood. Mother and I were featured in some of Dad's black-and-white images of this period, when he used us to show the perspective of people in the vast landscape. The Colorado River, the Grand Canyon, Marble Canyon, and Monument Valley were like home to me, and these worlds of rock and time have continued to call to me throughout my life. By showing me so much of the country on our photo trips, my parents taught me a love of the landscape.

Dad put a camera in my hands when I was six. At twelve, I hiked the six miles to Rainbow Bridge for the first time by myself—a solo backcountry trek into undammed wild country. This was before Glen Canyon Dam was built, before Lake Powell could even be imagined. On another hike down to the confluence, I was fascinated with the muddy

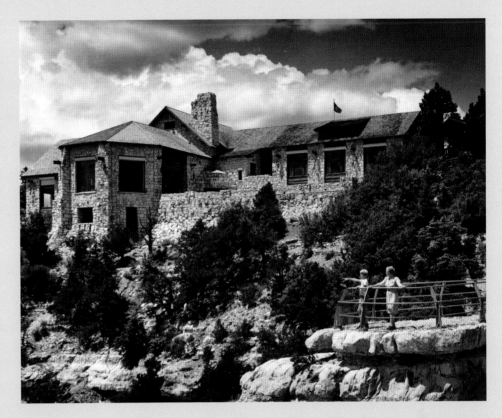

Colorado River, fluctuating enormously with seasonal runoff, meeting the turquoise waters of the Little Colorado. I remember the thrill of surprise and joy at my first glimpse of those braids of color deep in the canyon's heart. As I grew up, I developed a strong desire to see wild places for myself. I'd get an image of a place in my head and feel compelled to go there. Those early hikes, climbs, and river trips began for me a lifetime of outdoor adventure.

My father loved photographing the Grand Canyon and returned here throughout his life. A landscaper by profession, he was a self-taught photographer. I often served as his assistant, so I learned his trade of photography somewhat by osmosis. By my teens, I was well aware of the kind of photographs that would sell in the new market for landscape photographs in magazines,

calendars, and books, and of the cost to produce fine art prints. I was just out of high school when my parents loaned me their Ford station wagon to drive to Arizona to photograph the Grand Canyon by myself. Stopping in Las Vegas on the way, wowed by the bright lights and glittering people, I used up most of my 4x5 film. When I finally reached the canyon's North Rim, I took four shots at remote Toroweap Overlook. My father was furious that I'd wasted expensive film in Las Vegas, but my four shots at Toroweap hooked me on that precipitous drop to the river far below. I've braved the rough road to the dry campground and the hike out to Toroweap with my equipment many times over the years. One of my first published photographs was made there, an example of my commercially successful work at the time.

In the early 1950s, my father took me to the offices of *Arizona Highways*. Editor Raymond Carlson, with whom my father worked, said he'd publish a picture of mine as soon as I'd made a decent exposure. I was just eighteen when my first image for the magazine, of saguaro cactus, was used on the January 1955 cover. At that time there were just a few photographers doing Western landscape that inspired me—my dad, Ansel Adams, Ray Atkeson, and Ray Manley. They excelled in the commercial market opening up in response to post-World War II families eager to travel the scenic West. I was the next generation and jumped into this work with enthusiasm: not only Arizona, which I loved and photographed continuously, but all over the West and the entire National Park System. I was open to working spontaneously and creatively with my cumbersome 4x5 equipment, the state-of-the-art at the time. I captured moments in the great landscape as fast I could, wherever I could.

I brought my own children, Marc and Zandria, to the Grand Canyon when they were very young. They learned from me much as I had learned from my father. I put cameras in their hands early on during our many adventures. They learned how to see, feel, and make great images of their own. It's no surprise they both became photographers with their own professional specialties. ❖

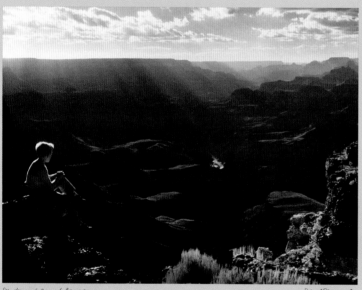

Mystery of Grand Canyon   *Josef Muench*

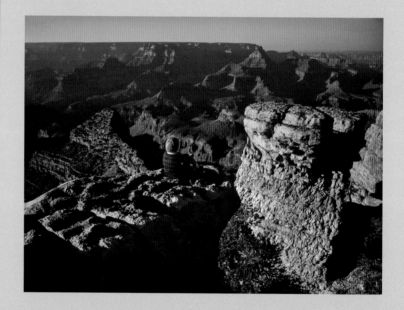

Above: My father, Josef Muench, made this photograph of me looking out over the Grand Canyon at Lipan Point about 1946. At ten years old, I had already been on many adventures in the park with my parents. PHOTO BY JOSEF MUENCH

Above right: I photographed my son, Marc Muench, at the South Rim in 1976.

Facing page: The rimrock at Mather Point on the South Rim is one place I have looked for "natural connections" as I scout with my camera for the most intriguing forms and light.

Natural Connections

I have returned to Grand Canyon National Park in every season for most of my life. Many of the photographs I've made here have been published. But I will always seek new ways to show my fascination with the canyon's secrets. I look for unusual conditions, the promise of storm clouds, or a first snow. I look for ways to be in the right place at the right time every time I visit the Grand Canyon. Conditions that lead me to a good image might drive most visitors inside: a coming storm, a rising fog, a steep hike, a long wait.

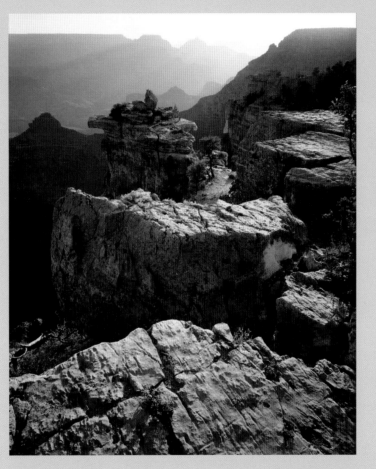

I need to spend time seeing for myself what might happen at a particular location. Then, I look for what I call "natural connections." It might be a detail right at my feet that becomes my subject, with the landscape in the background. I evolved this way of seeing over time, until the way I connect with a subject became the signature of my work. I wanted to look through these natural connections I discovered in the field, to let them become part of the way I see, to let changing light define the image I make. In these moments I connect myself with the special qualities of the place around me, beyond me, and beneath my feet. Through making a photograph, I'm connecting with myself, and with what intrigues me.

I have a passion for seeking the "timeless moment," that slice of time between then and now when my camera shutter stops time. Photography represents the past meeting the future in the now—when that one moment becomes eternal. A photographic image represents a memory, closely tied to my sensory impressions of a place. Done well, that one shutter click allows me to glimpse back into the whole story that so intrigued me.

I find the Grand Canyon's forms and foregrounds as thrilling as its famous wide vistas. I'm fascinated by form versus light and contrast—where my eye goes. I force my equipment to work in new ways to make the images I visualize. I might photograph landscapes with a telephoto lens to emphasize form, or hone right in on a group of cobbles under a running stream. I look for ways to show the unexpected, the unusual frame that defines the feeling of a place.

The power in this forbidding, intimidating landscape challenges me. And yet on each visit here I find more of the Grand Canyon's beauty in its rock forms—in its exposed layers lying open like a book. The more I learned about the rock layers here—Coconino, Kaibab, Moenkopi, Redwall Limestone—the more they came alive

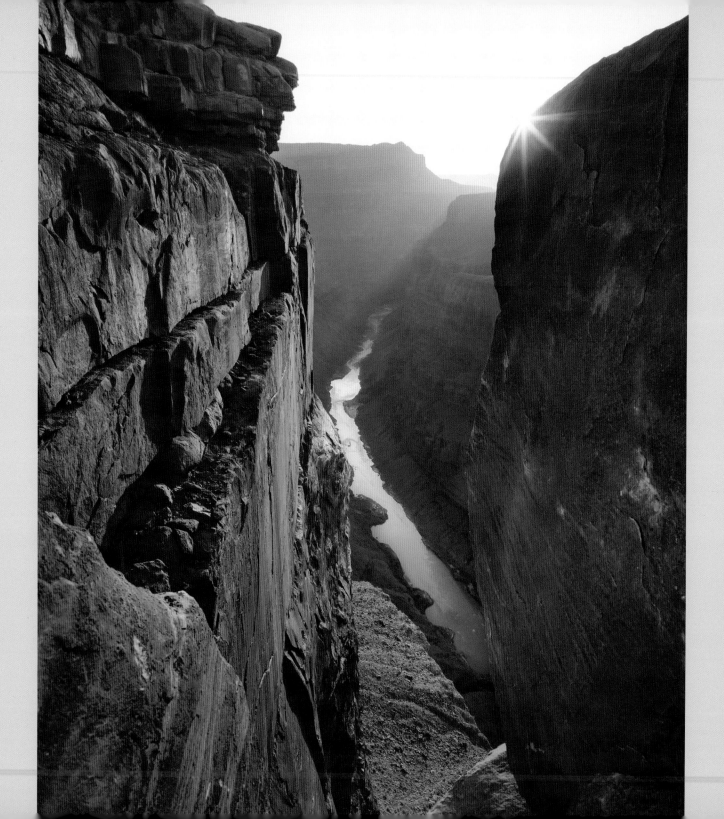

to me. I think of them as poetry in time. In winter the slots at Toroweap, looking east as the rising sun warms the rock, tell me a compelling story of rock light and stone time. By June, I find amazing light at dawn on the ribbon-like river below and still avoid sun flares. I work with the seasons, the weather, and the conditions of the day and revise my plans in the moment. Good timing helps me expose for that elusive backlit quality that will tell the story of the Grand Canyon's layers in time. A glint of the river suggests hidden mysteries from the past.

Floating the Colorado River through Grand Canyon National Park has been integral to my knowing this great place. My first assignment trip down the river, with writer David Toll in 1969, was part of a commemorative article on the John Wesley Powell Expedition for *Arizona Highways*. Powell had always been a hero of mine. That unstoppable one-armed Civil War veteran and his wonderful accounts of the river canyon inspired me to keep going on many steep canyon hikes, or for tricky tripod setups on the very edge of the rim. What would Powell have seen that I could capture now to bring this deep canyon's sights and sounds to life on the pages of a magazine? In those days I carried a Linhof 4x5 and tripod everywhere, including on the river trip. I hiked up Deer Creek Canyon with my gear as fast as I could to make some waterfall images, then

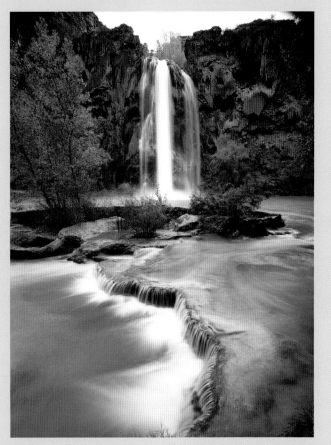

raced back to the waiting boats. David Toll and I also hiked up to the South Rim late one day for dinner at El Tovar, then hustled back down the trail to the river at midnight to sleep on a sandbar near Bright Angel Creek. It was a memorable adventure, like all journeys down the canyon.

On the river, views in every direction have their own power. I remember well the dramatic moment of looking up at Toroweap from the brink of Lava Falls. There is hardly a more timeless moment than each split second as another boat makes it through the rapid. In each instant the roaring river showed me how it carved the rock world of the deep inner gorge over time.

Each time I approach Grand Canyon, I experience the physical sensation of this great chasm. A mile below the rims, the separate world of the Colorado River beckons with its rock-carving red water, winding side canyons, and lush waterfalls. Hiking to Havasu Canyon's incredible turquoise waters has been one of my favorite side trips over the decades.

The Grand Canyon is a marvel of geology and hydrology, and a tantalizing challenge to photograph in all seasons. The bold wildness of this place, its near inaccessibility

Above: I hiked down the canyon from the village on Havasupai tribal lands to photograph Havasu Falls' incredible turquoise water in motion.

Facing page: At sunrise, the red rock slabs at Toroweap East Overlook frame my view of the river gleaming below.

at times, has always been part of its allure. Hiking out to a remote location, quite alone with my thoughts and feelings, I see the Grand Canyon's drama in new ways with each visit.

Over time I have photographed some of the iconic views of Grand Canyon National Park decades apart. Rock may seem timeless when I am making a photograph, but wind and weather constantly reshape the fine details. Junipers I have foregrounded have completed their life cycles; ephemeral cactus flowers bloom (or not) depending on rainfall. Every snowmelt moves and re-shapes tiny cracks. Rains can turn dry side canyons into rushing flash flood channels. Tributaries to the river contribute to carving deep within the canyon, resulting in visual changes each decade at classic destinations like Elves Chasm. If I look closely at images I've taken decades apart at the same site, I can revisit and relive a sequence of timeless moments. The shapes and forms of rock and water, continually rearranging in geologic time, are, for me, the greatest gift of the Grand Canyon landscape.

In summer, the long driving distances between the Grand Canyon's North and South Rims can seem endless to me, the intense heat in the bottom of the canyon unknowable from the rims. I often spend time on the North Rim in autumn when the colors and shadows are incredibly inspiring and the moments of changing light pass so very quickly. I might hike down to the canyon's river heart in February or March, when I start out in snow at the top, and the canyon's geology reveals itself with changes in light and shadow. I never run out of sub-jects at the Grand Canyon, even from the spots I've photographed many times. ❖

Above: I made this image of water-carved rock at Elves Chasm in 1966. The contrast between huge tumbled boulders and the delicate stream of water over moss and fern has captured my imagination on every river trip I have taken down the Grand Canyon's inner gorge.

Facing page: A similar composition of Elves Chasm, taken several decades later in 1997, shows me the change in plant life by the waterfall over time.

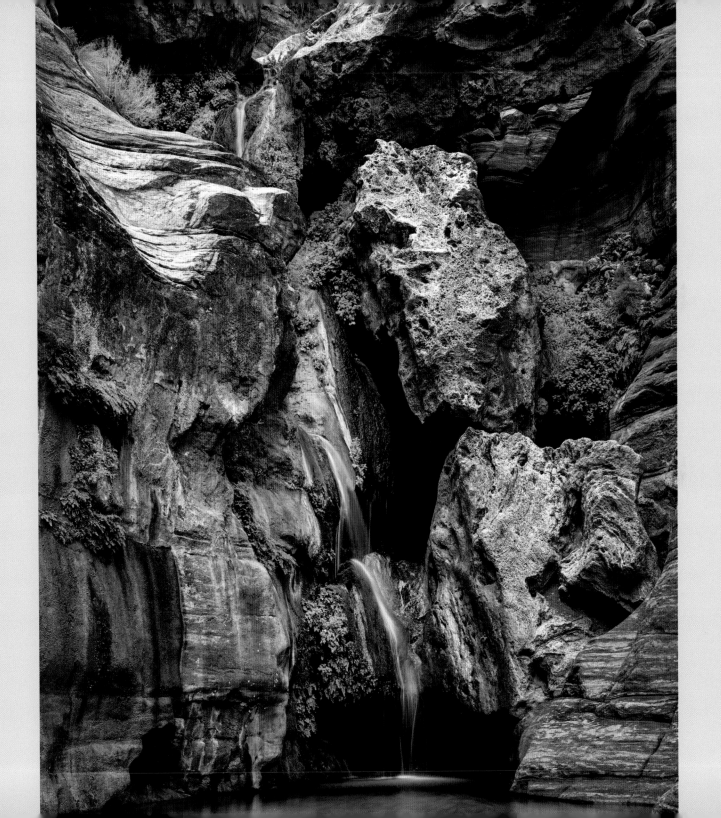

13

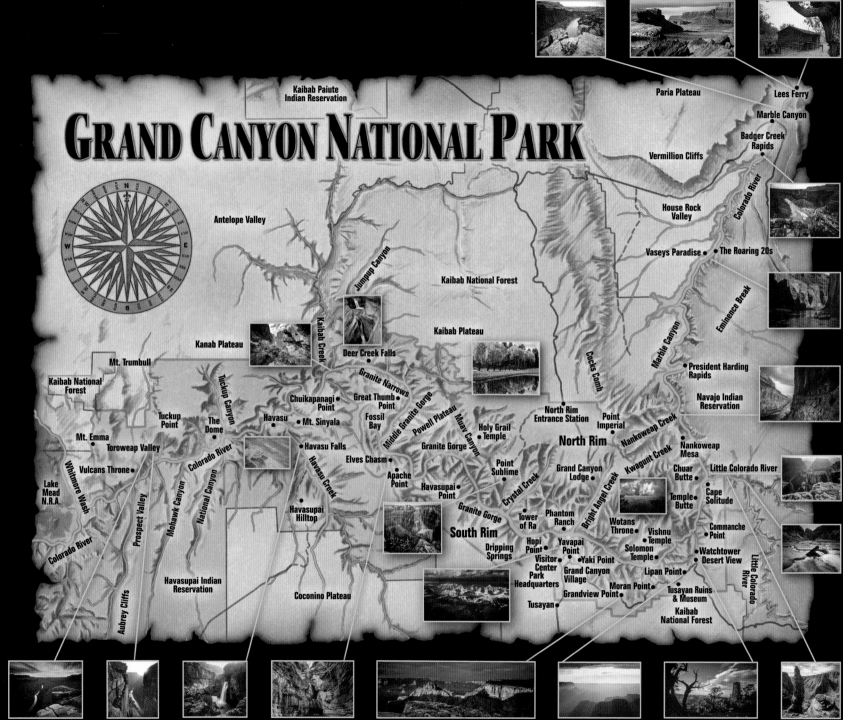

GRAND CANYON NATIONAL PARK

Kaibab Paiute Indian Reservation

Paria Plateau

Lees Ferry

Marble Canyon

Badger Creek Rapids

Vermillion Cliffs

Antelope Valley

House Rock Valley

Colorado River

Vaseys Paradise · The Roaring 20s

Jumpup Canyon

Kaibab National Forest

Eminence Break

Kaibab Creek

Kaibab Plateau

Deer Creek Falls

Marble Canyon

Cocks Comb

President Harding Rapids

Kanab Plateau

Navajo Indian Reservation

Mt. Trumbull

Granite Narrows

Great Thumb Point

Kaibab National Forest

Tuckup Canyon

Chuikapanagi Point

Middle Granite Gorge

Powell Plateau

North Rim Entrance Station

Point Imperial

Nankoweap Creek

Nankoweap Mesa

Tuckup Point

The Dome

Havasu

Mt. Sinyala

Fossil Bay

Granite Gorge

Muav Canyon

Holy Grail Temple

North Rim

Chuar Butte

Little Colorado River

Mt. Emma

Toroweap Valley

Havasu Falls

Elves Chasm

Point Sublime

Grand Canyon Lodge

Kwagunt Creek

Temple Butte

Cape Solitude

Vulcans Throne

Colorado River

Apache Point

Havasupai Point

Crystal Creek

Bright Angel Creek

Wotans Throne

Vishnu Temple

Commanche Point

Lake Mead N.R.A.

Mohawk Canyon

National Canyon

Havasu Creek

Granite Gorge

Tower of Ra

Phantom Ranch

Solomon Temple

Watchtower Desert View

Lipan Point

Colorado River

Prospect Valley

Havasupai Hilltop

South Rim

Dripping Springs

Hopi Point

Yavapai Point

Grand Canyon Village

Moran Point

Tusayan Ruins & Museum

Little Colorado River

Aubrey Cliffs

Whitmore Wash

Visitor Center Park Headquarters

Yaki Point

Grandview Point

Kaibab National Forest

Havasupai Indian Reservation

Coconino Plateau

Tusayan

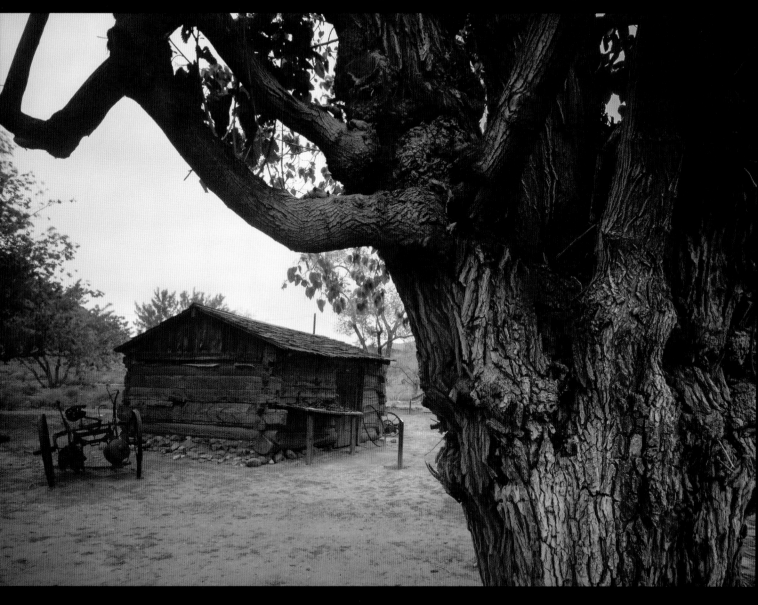

Above: An old cottonwood frames the historic cabin at Lees Ferry.

Facing page: Map of David Muench's photographic journey of "timeless moments" through Grand Canyon National Park.

Right: The old gauging station downstream from Lees Ferry, with the Vermillion Cliffs rising in the background, is one of the sights river runners see as they begin journeys through the Grand Canyon. This image reminds me of placid floats on the Colorado River and the thrills of rapids to come.

Below: An ephemeral rain pool reflects the water-carved rock layers in Cathedral Canyon, near Lees Ferry.

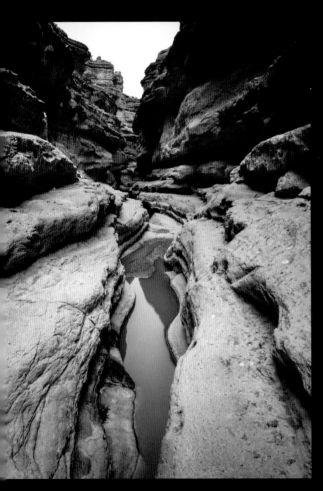

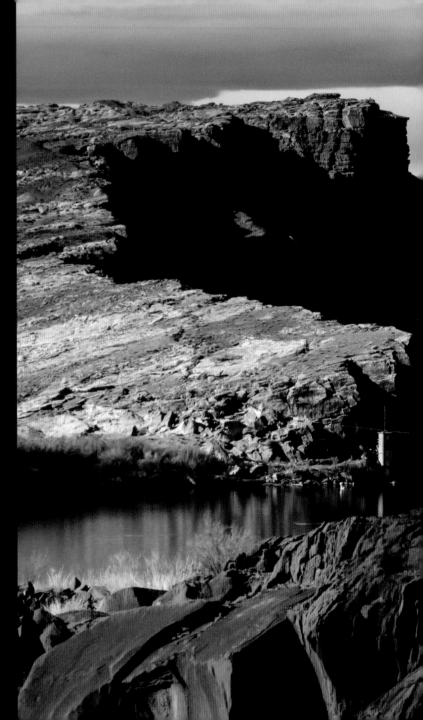

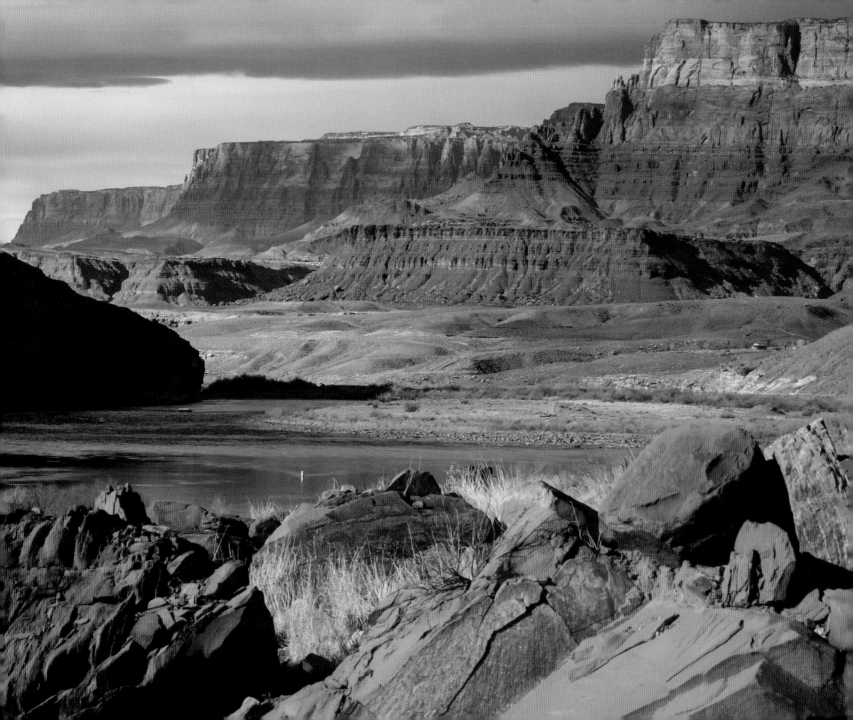

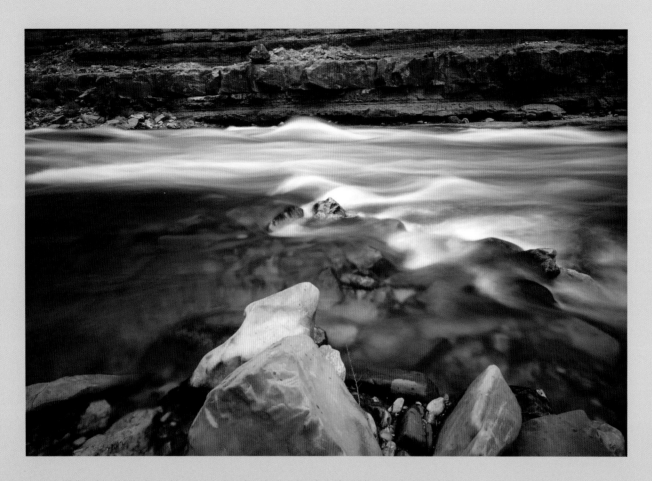

Above: Whitewater rushes where side canyons deposit rock along the river. I found these rock shapes in the Colorado River downstream from Lees Ferry in Marble Canyon. They intrigued me with their momentary stability against the blur of the water.

Right: A beavertail cactus blooms on rimrock above the river, a great example of my search for foreground elements to dramatize the river view upstream in Marble Canyon.

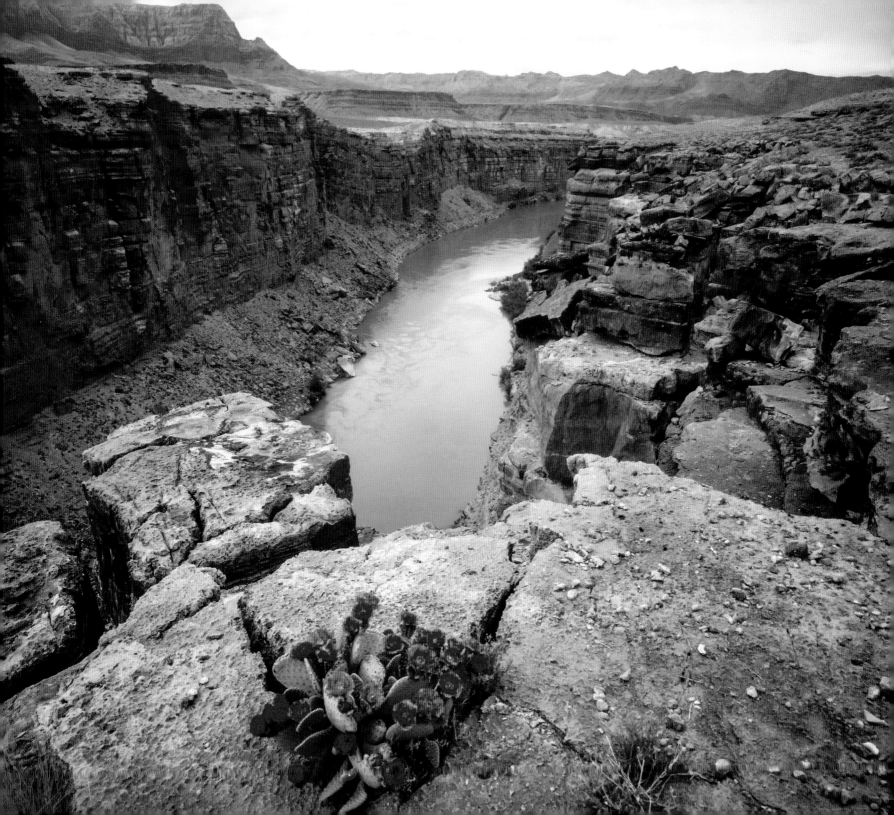

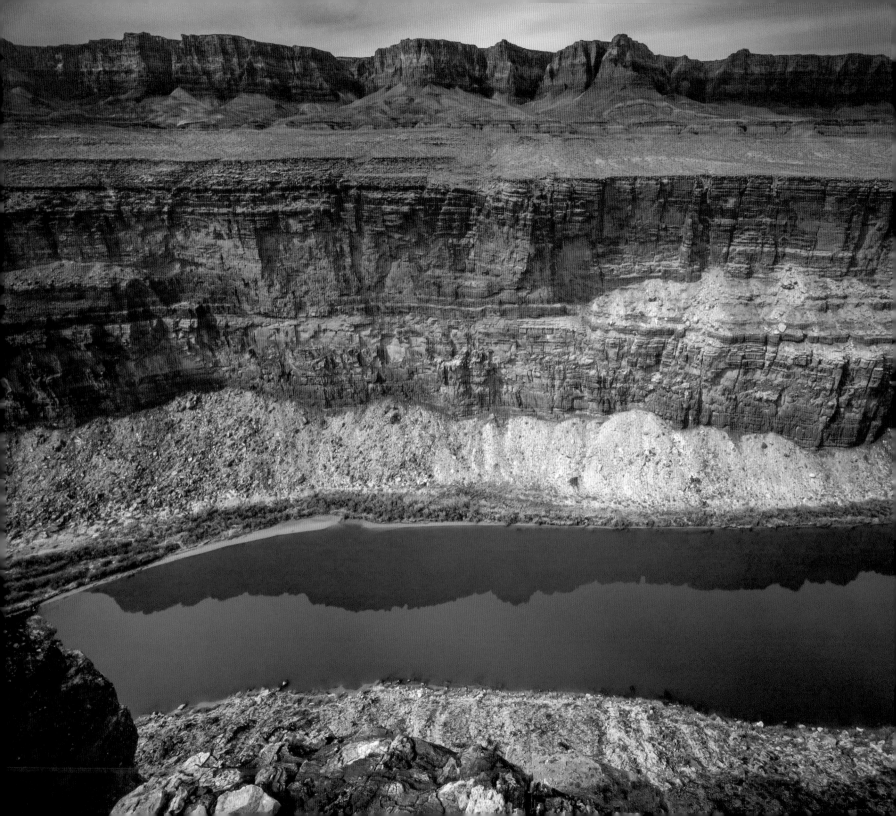

Left: When I climbed up to look across the many layers of time in the rock carved by the Colorado River in Marble Canyon, I was captivated by the shadow of the cliffs on the inviting deep green water.

Below: I looked for a window view of the river below, and found this sheltered cave in the cliff above.

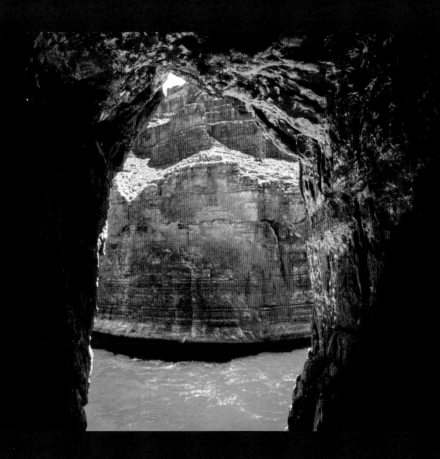

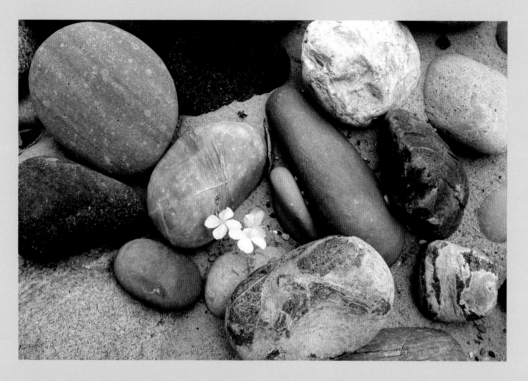

Above: Colorful river rock cobbles, strewn along the riverside, shelter a delicate primrose bloom emerging straight up out of the fine sands.

Right: I found this high rimrock view looking downstream over Badger Rapids in Marble Canyon, and made this graphic study of the rock deposits from eroding side canyons.

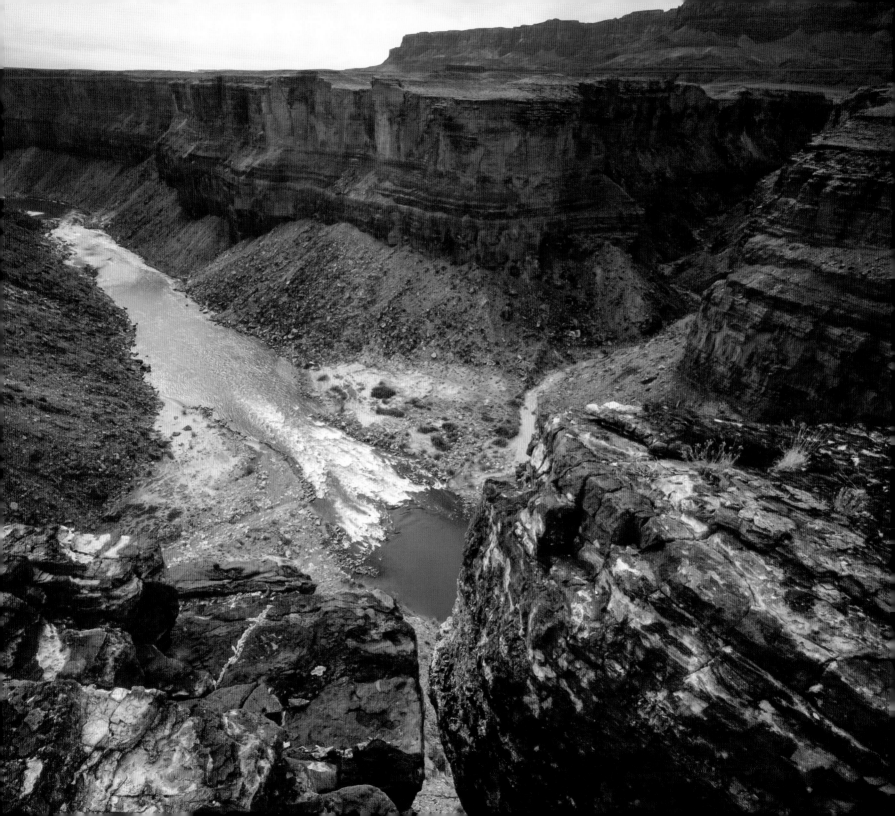

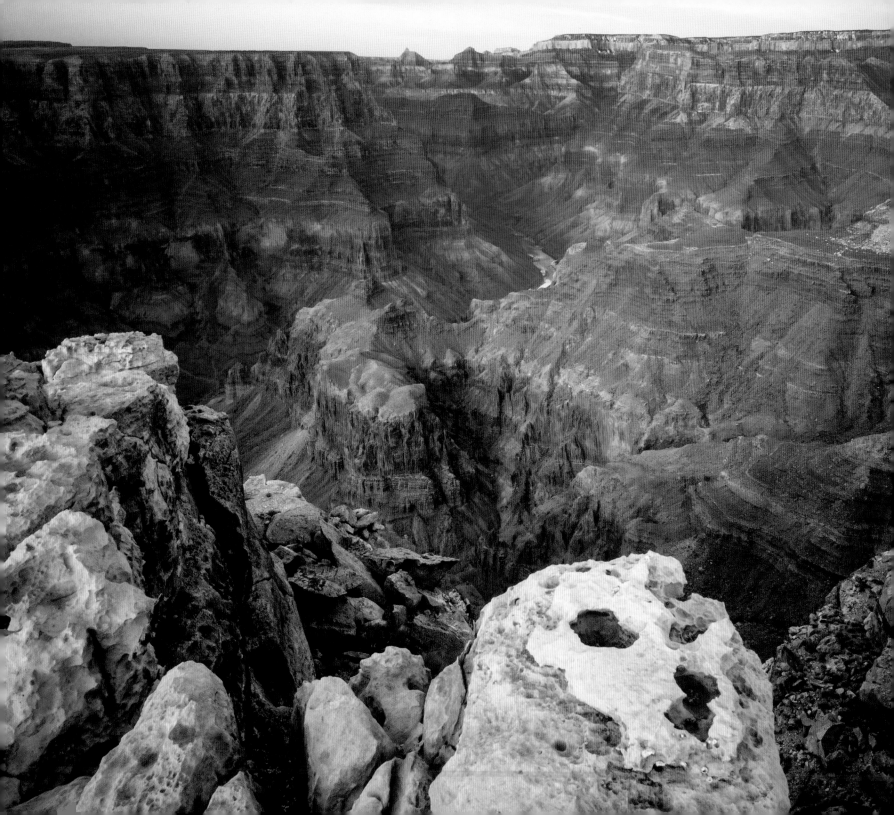

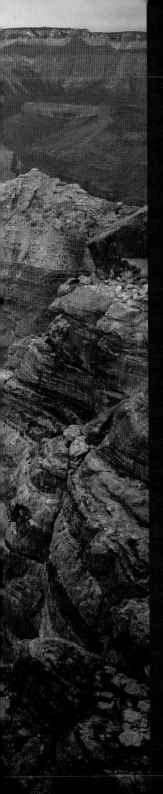

Left: From the rimrock I could see glimpses of the Little Colorado and Colorado Rivers above their confluence. Dawn light accents Chuar Butte and the North Rim in the far distance.

Below: Morning light just touches the canyon wall at Nankoweap, Marble Canyon.

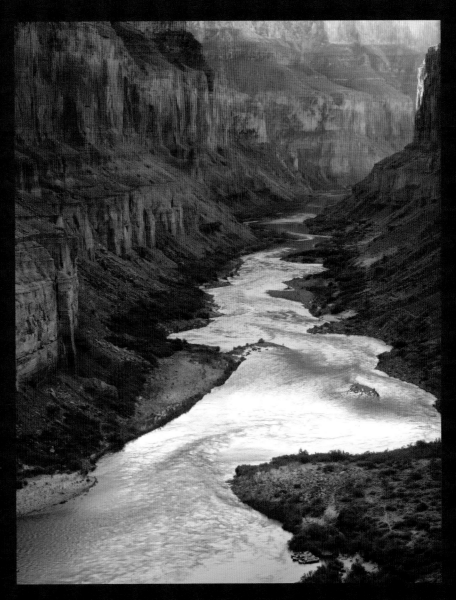

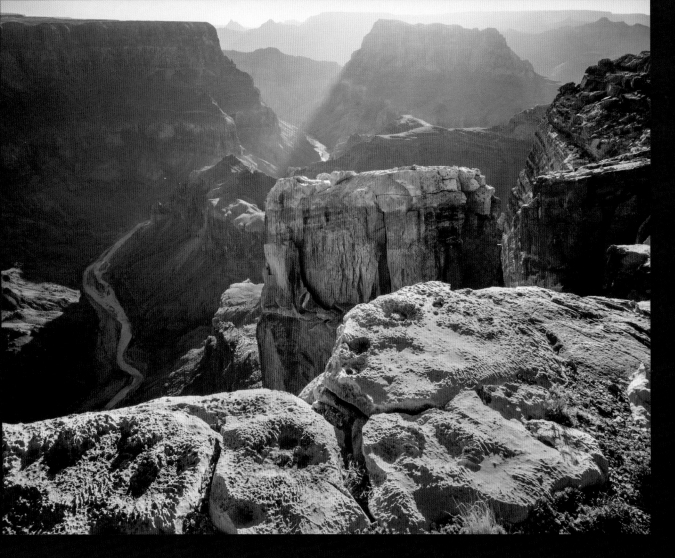

Above: The Little Colorado River flows toward its confluence with the mighty Colorado deep in Marble Canyon. Cape Solitude rises to the left of backlit Chuar Butte, with the two merged rivers flowing between them.

Facing page: Jagged rimrock caught my eye from Tatahatso Point. Over time the Colorado River carved

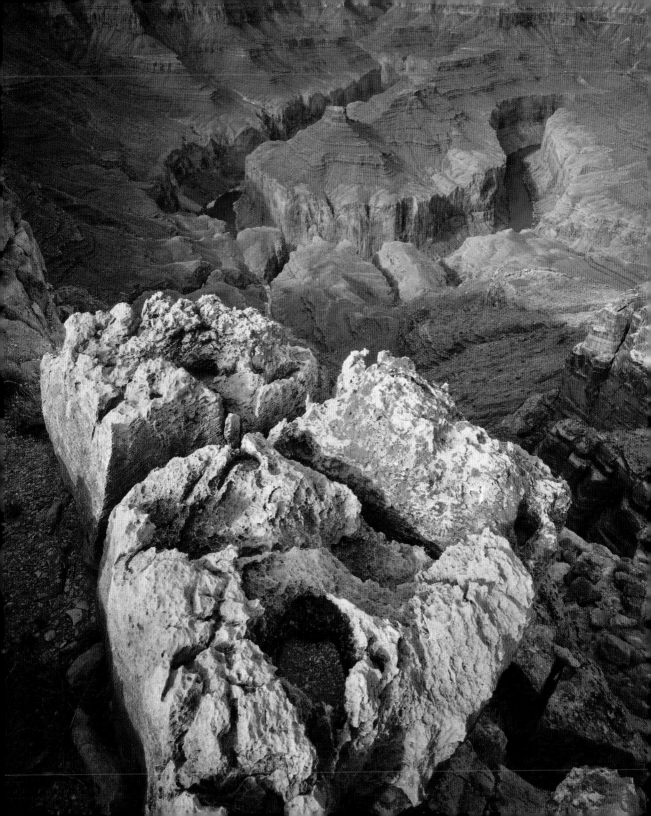

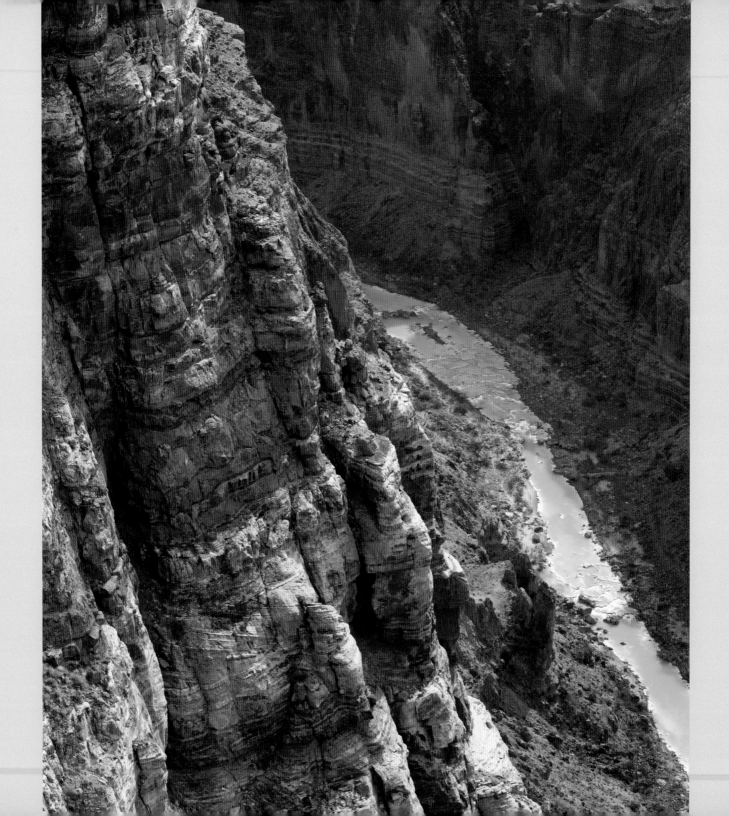

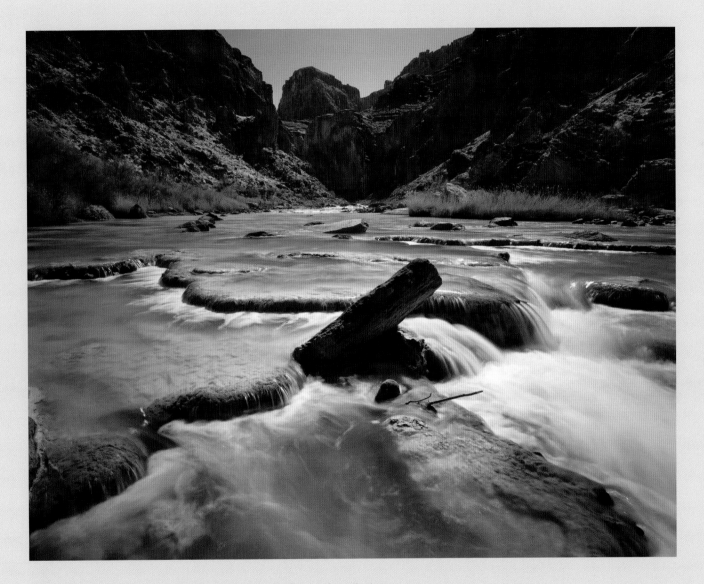

Above: The Little Colorado River's distinctive turquoise waters flow over travertine terraces.

Facing page: High above the Little Colorado River, I lingered for a moment on my steep hike down from the rim to the river with my 4x5 to photograph these colorful layers of rock. Then I kept descending to study the blue waters up close.

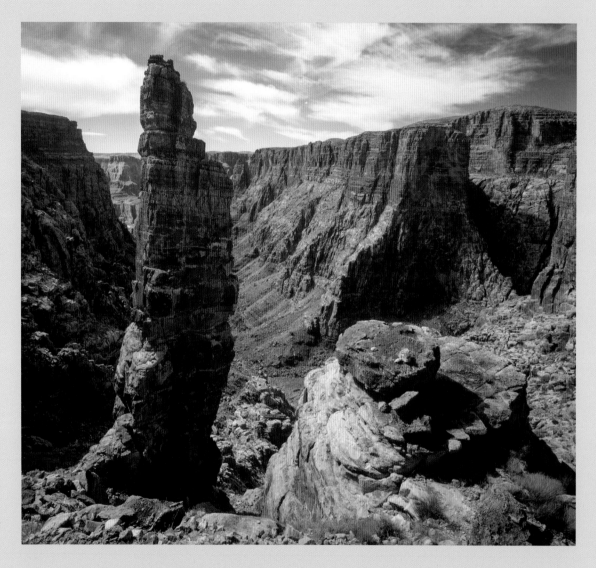

Above: Hiking between rim and river in search of intriguing compositions, I found this Coconino sandstone pinnacle and a tilted section of rim in the Little Colorado River canyon.

Right: Glorious autumn light inspired this image looking upriver from Comanche Point to the confluence of the Colorado and Little Colorado Rivers in Marble Canyon. Deep shadows highlight the eroded slopes of Temple and Chuar Buttes.

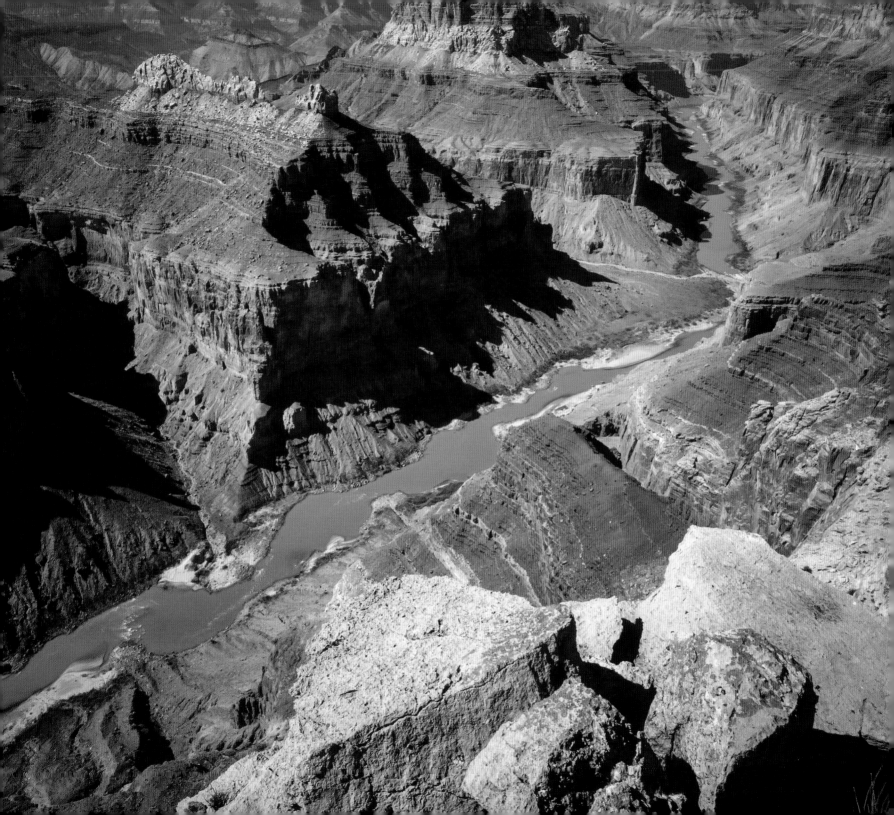

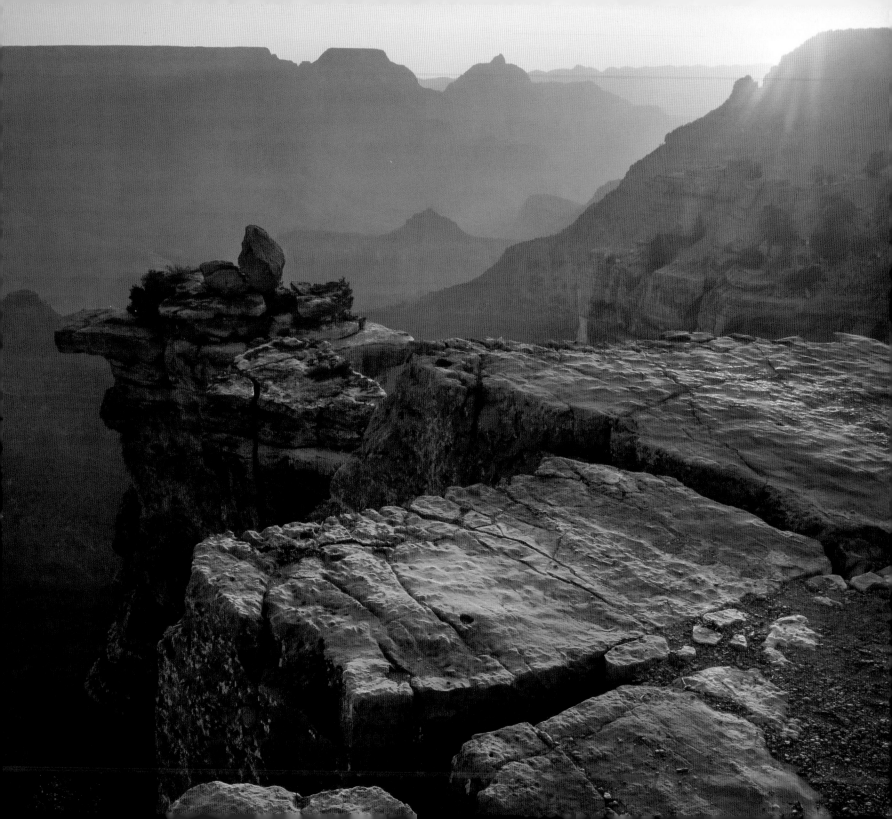

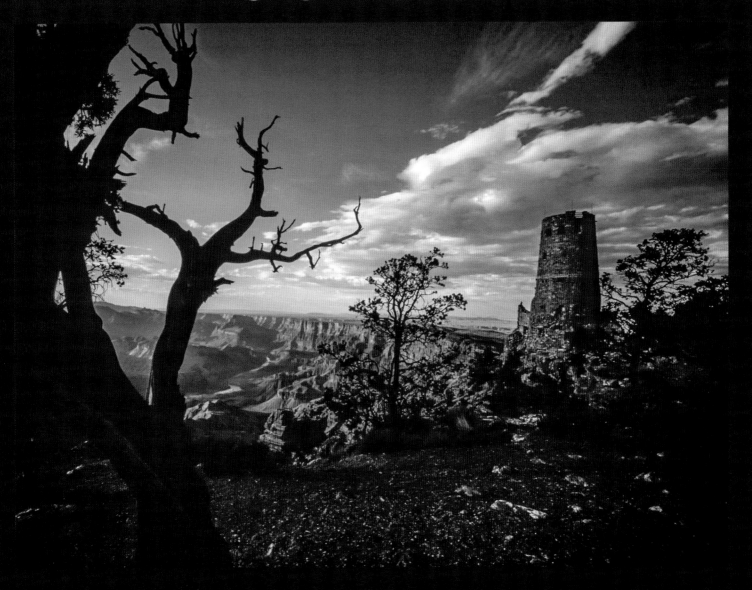

Above: On the South Rim, Desert View's Watchtower and a rugged juniper frame the Colorado River at sunset in late winter. The first Grand Canyon viewpoint from the East Entrance, Desert View Point is one of my favorite places to walk out along the rim and experience the great abyss.

Facing page: On a cold spring morning at Desert View, the first rays of sun define the rimrock shapes before me.

Right: Evening storm light in February near Yavapai Point inspired this study of light, shadow, and color on the iconic Temple formations.

Below: This telephoto V-cut image through Kaibab Limestone near Desert View frames a long view of canyon rock.

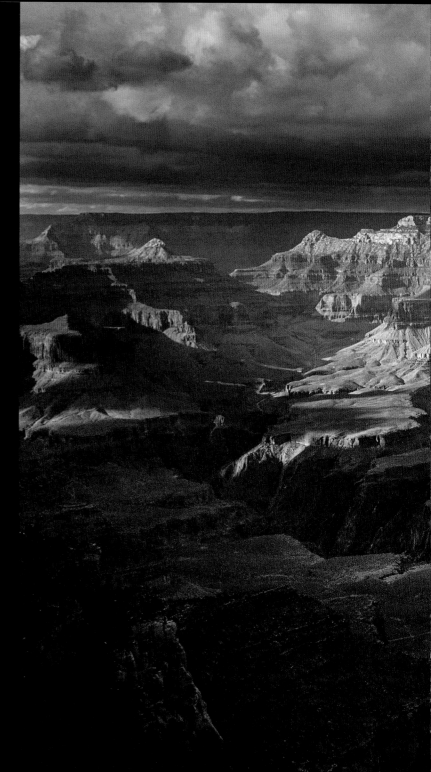

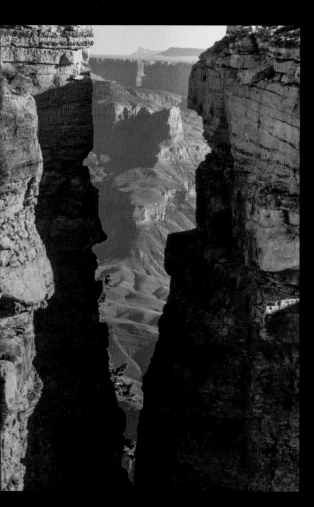

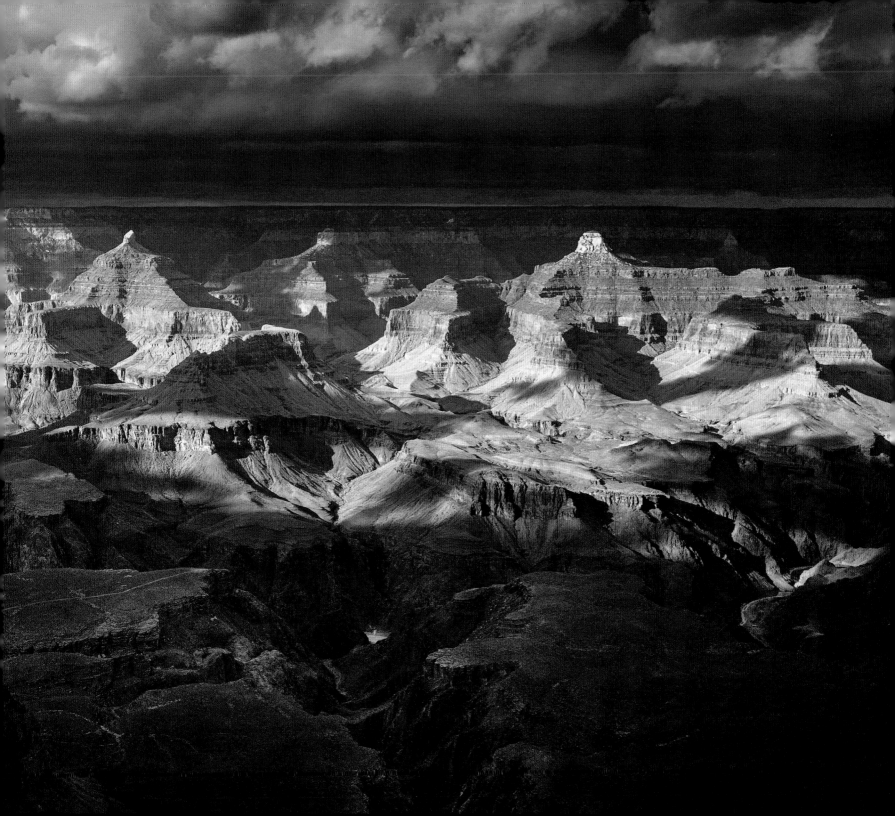

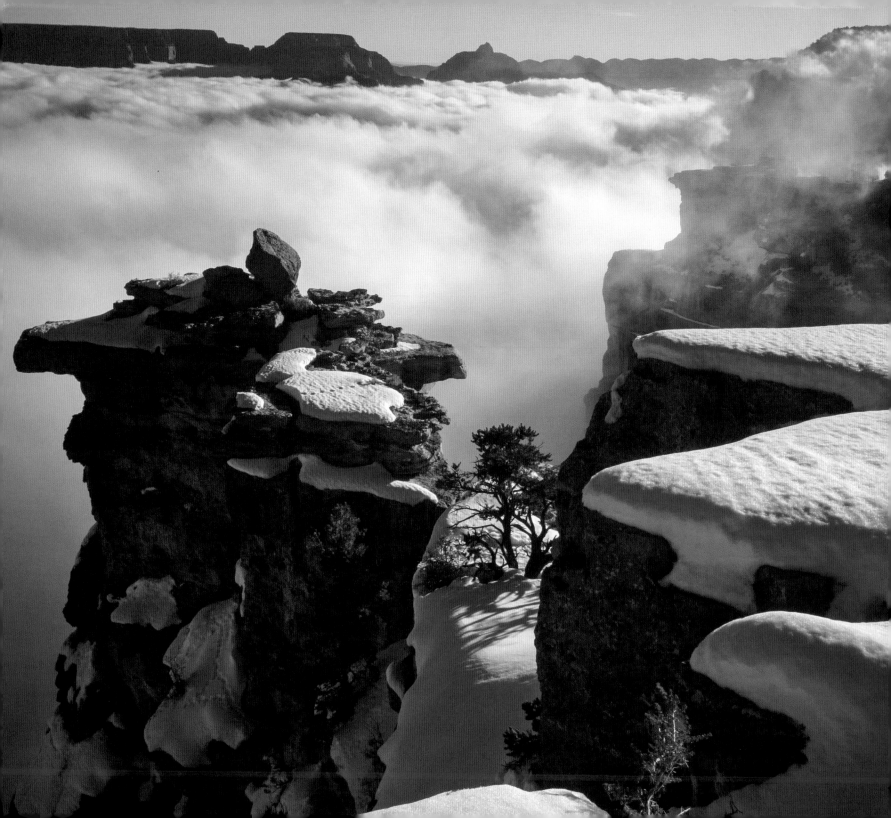

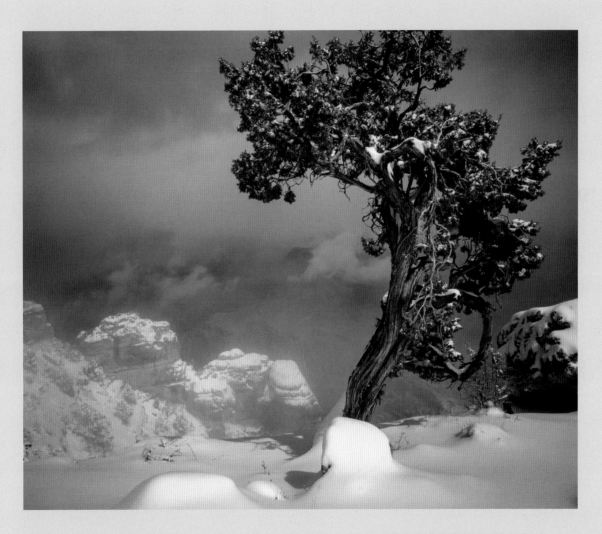

Above: Fresh morning snow highlights the shaggy trunk and thick needles of a juniper on the South Rim. Winter storm clouds drift over the North Rim.

Left: Cape Royal, Wotans Throne, and Vishnu Temple rise above winter fog before a coming storm. The rimrock near Mather Point offers a perspective of impossibly steep canyon walls in this image, yet animals have left tracks all over the rock peninsula.

Next pages: Late winter sunset light casts a shadow on Coronado Butte and the South Rim in this panorama taken from Grandview Point.

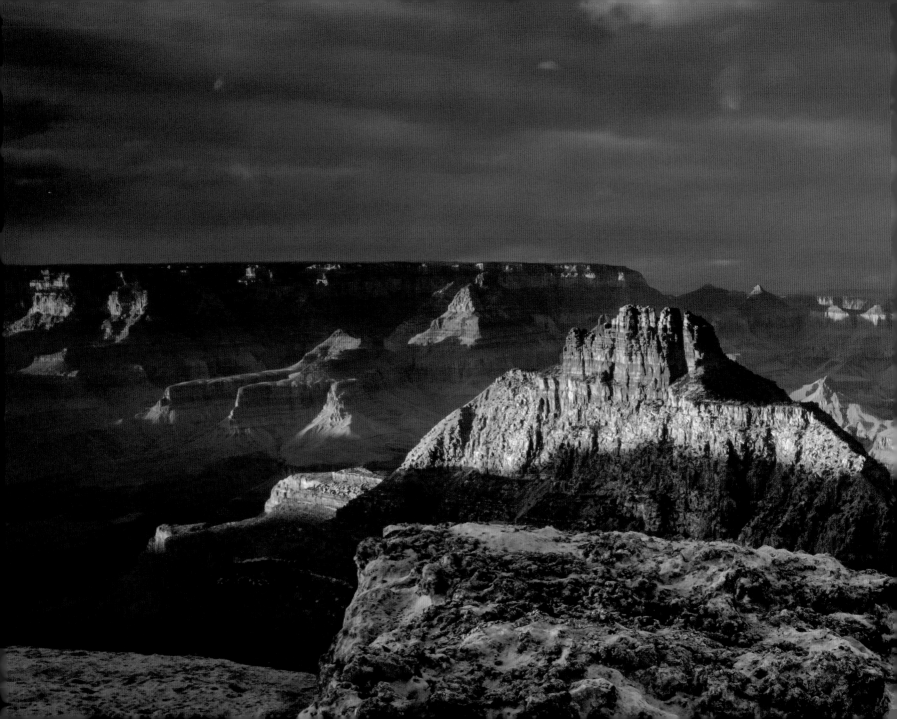

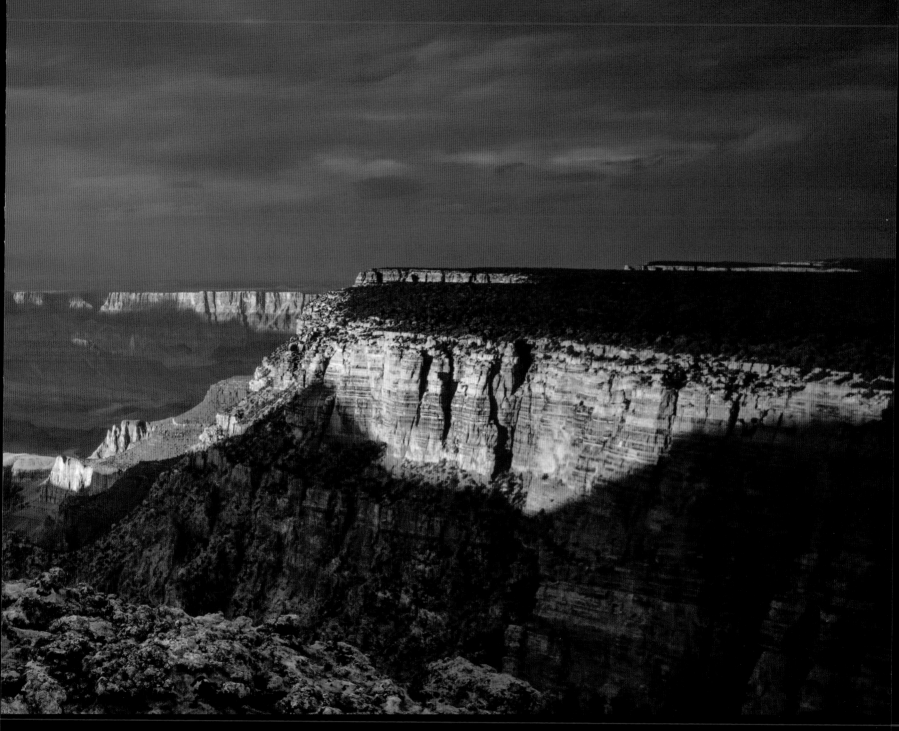

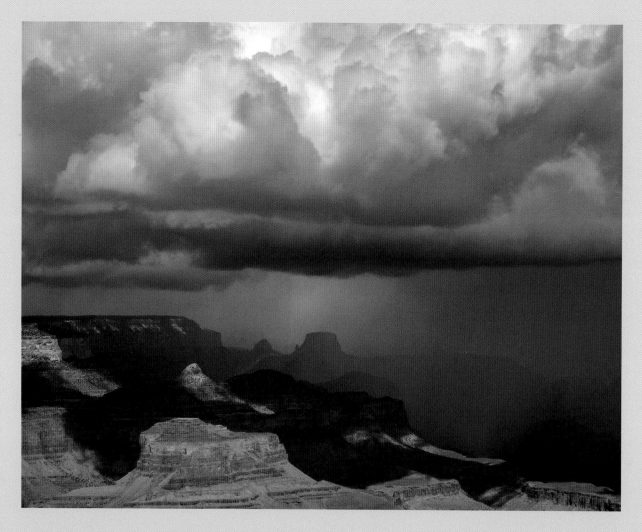

Above: From Navajo Point, I watched a winter storm drop rain and snow in the canyon before me while I braced my tripod on the windy rim.

Right: This image made on the same day at Desert View allowed me to play with the rock layers in the foreground, the distant river, and a fast-moving curtain of rain over the canyon in between.

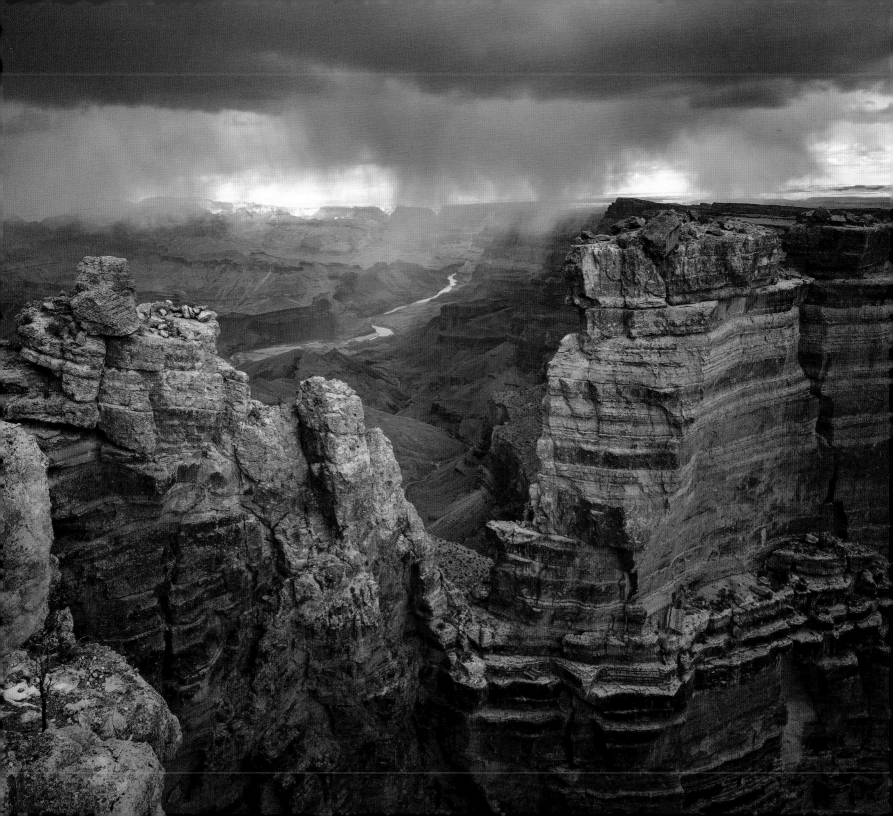

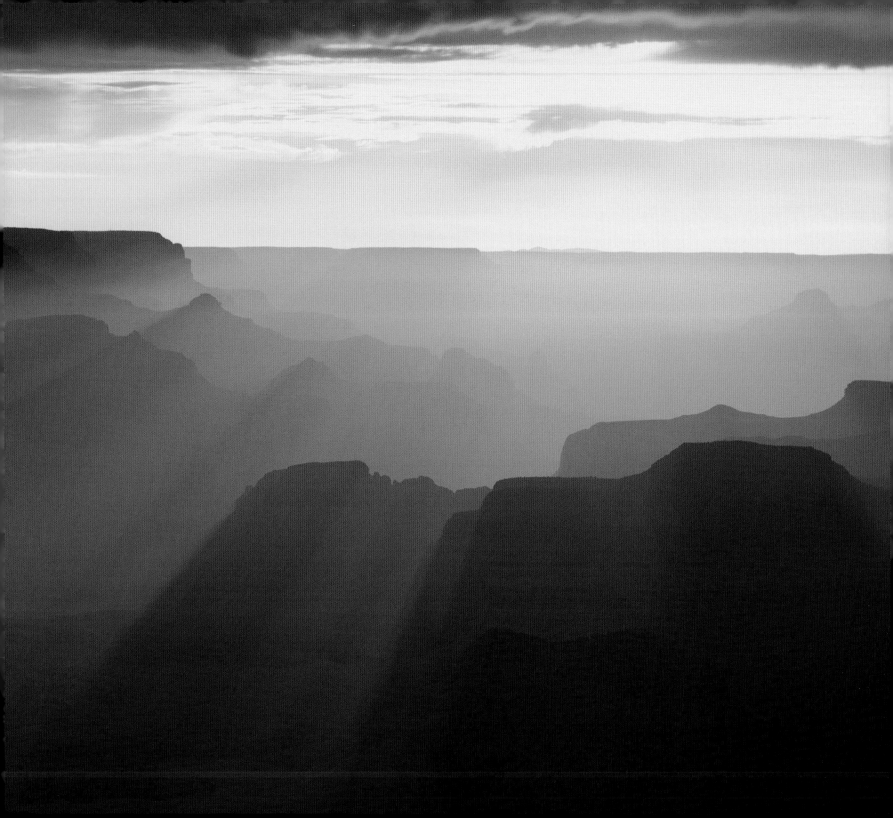

Left: Facing west from Lipan Point, sunset light flows directly toward me. Intense backlight softens the strong horizontal rock layers of the canyon.

Below: The defined edges of this limestone formation and rugged plant life on the rim contrast with the soft mauve and olive background ridges at sunrise.

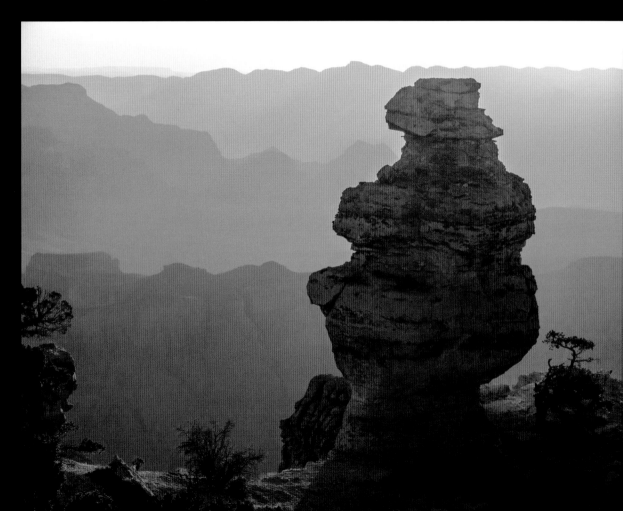

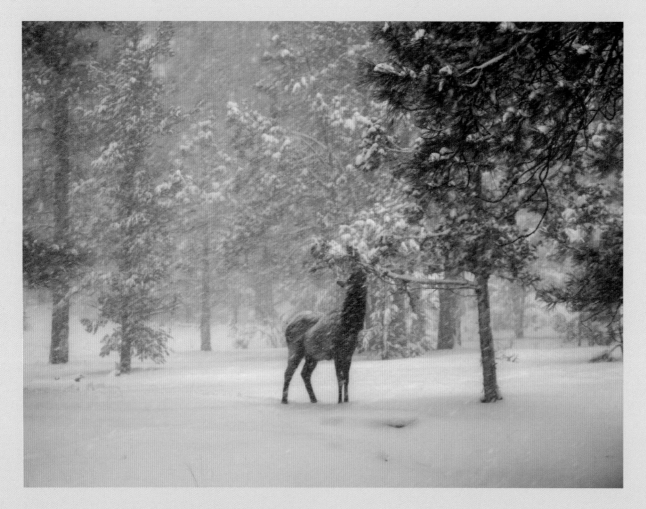

Above: In a snowstorm, my eye was drawn to the muscular shape of a cow elk reaching for ponderosa pine needles.

Right: A brief clearing in a winter storm brings sunlight and shadow to the snow-covered South Rim, with tantalizing glimpses of the clouds shrouding the canyon. I caught this timeless moment just before the wind changed the freshly fallen snow.

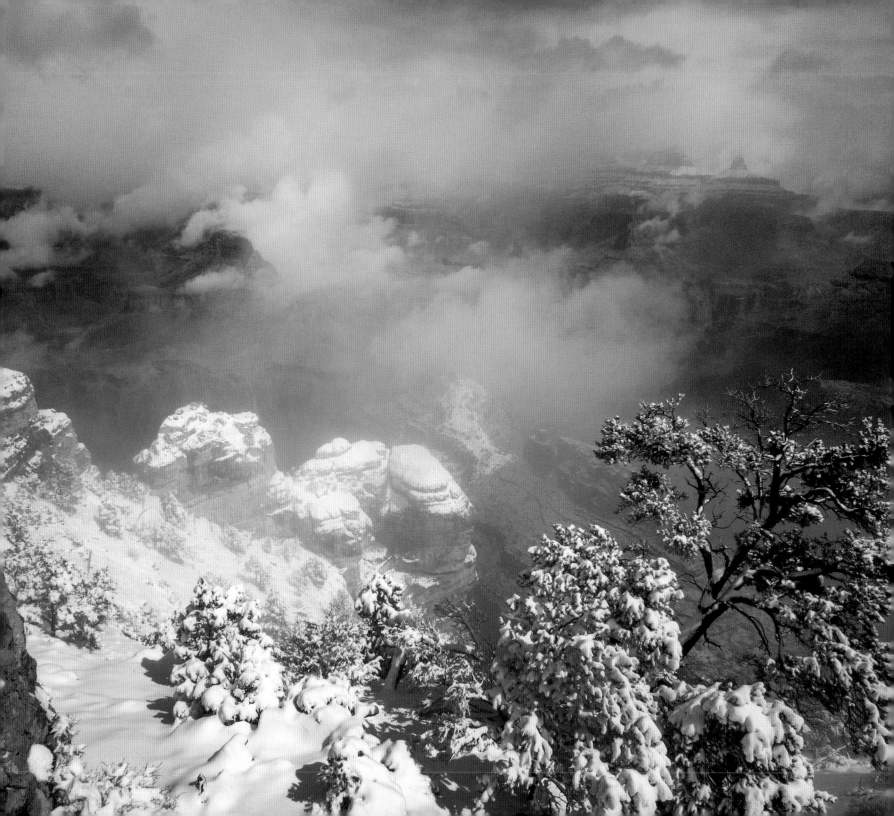

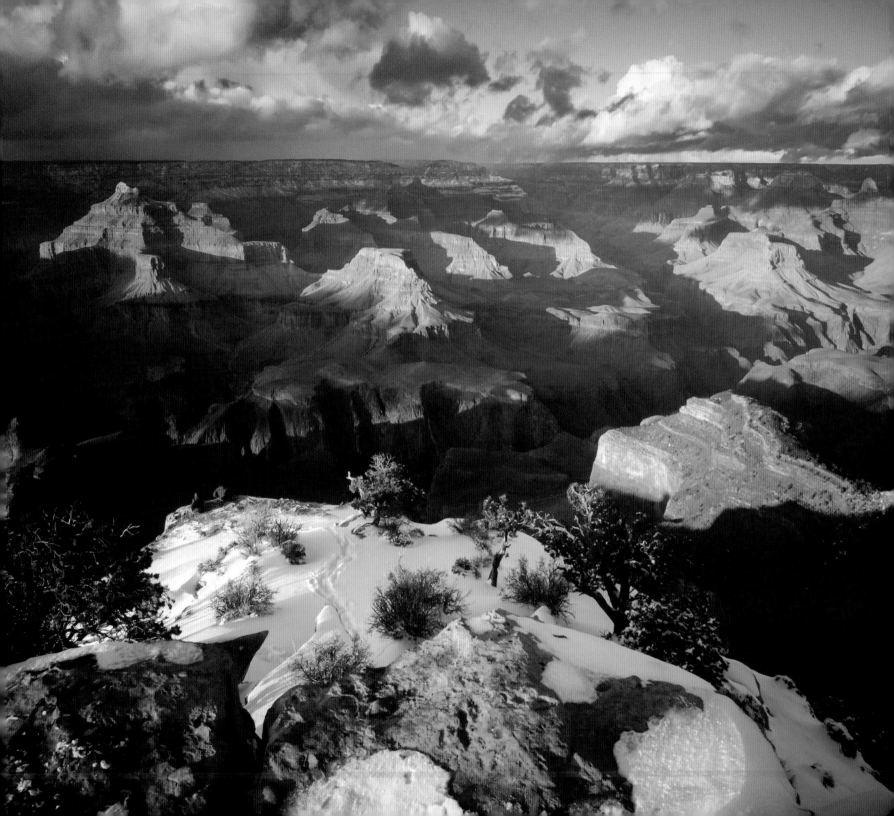

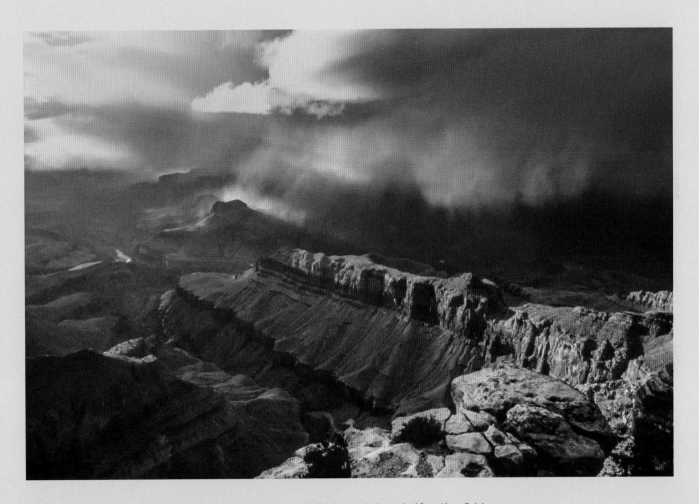

Above: A late afternoon rain shower passes beyond Escalante Butte in this image photographed from Lipan Point.

Facing page: On a winter afternoon at Powell Point, the Grand Canyon displays its rock temples in intense warm light and shadow. The North Rim in the distance, a thousand feet higher in elevation than the South Rim, is covered in heavy snow.

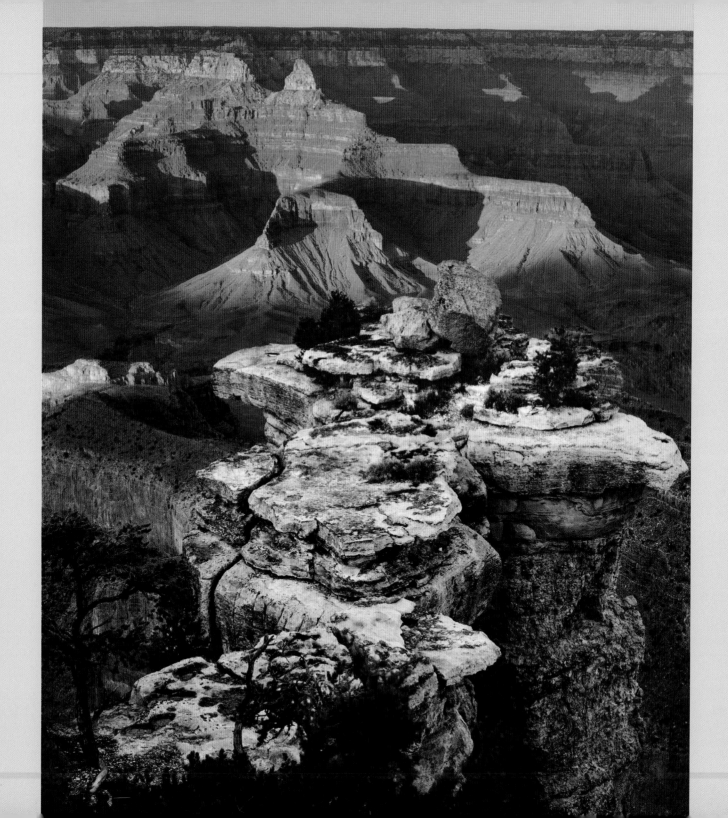

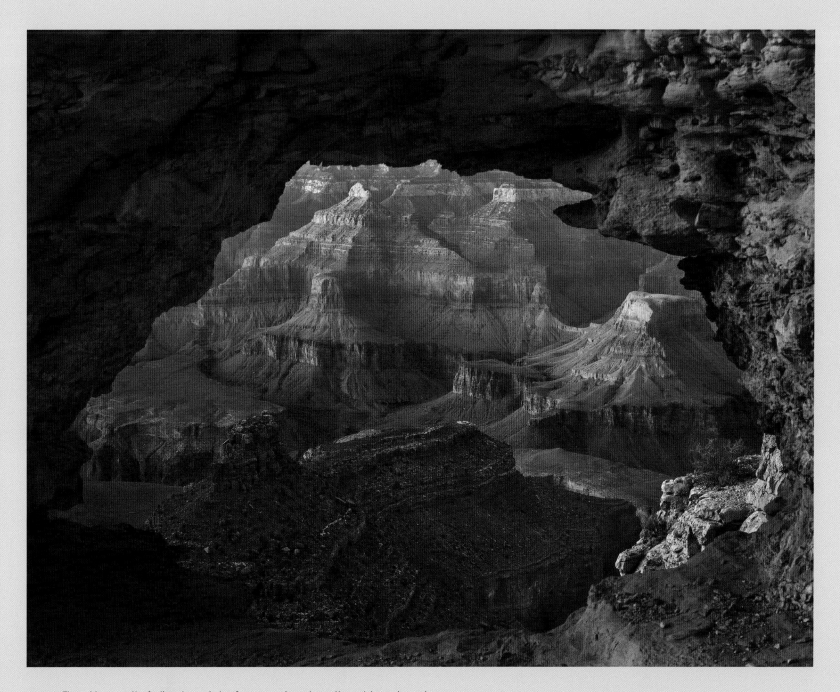

Above: The golden warmth of a limestone window frames evening color on the rock layers beyond.

Facing page: I waited for the winter evening's light and shadow on Brahma and Zoroaster Temples and Sumner Butte to make this image of an eroded rim feature at Yavapai Point.

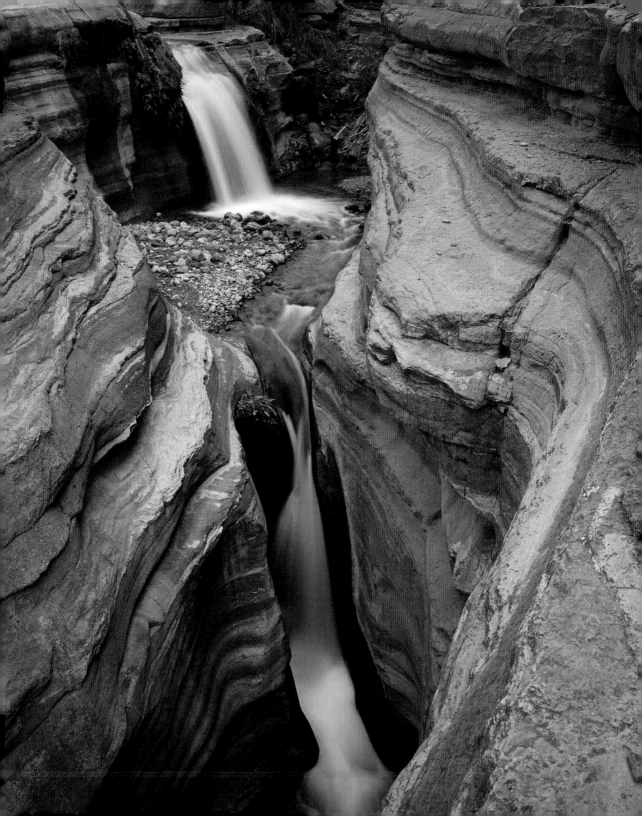

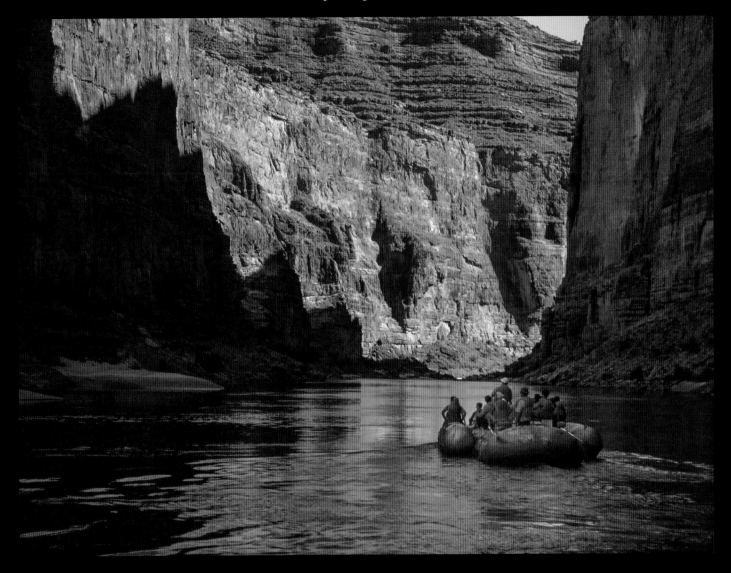

Above: On a peaceful stretch of the Colorado River, rafters float around a bend of brightly lit red walls. Late afternoon reflective light gave me that incandescent glow on the water.

Facing page: On one of my earliest river trips, I hiked above Deer Creek Gorge to see these ribbons of water and the rock walls they have carved over time.

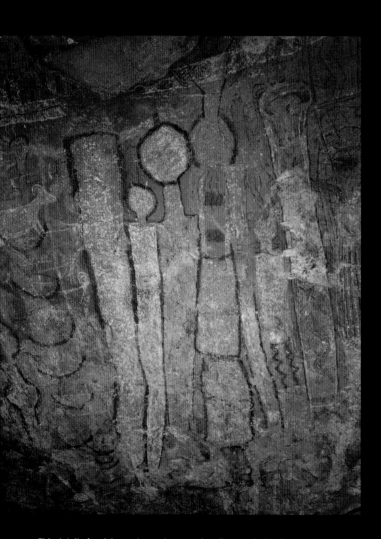

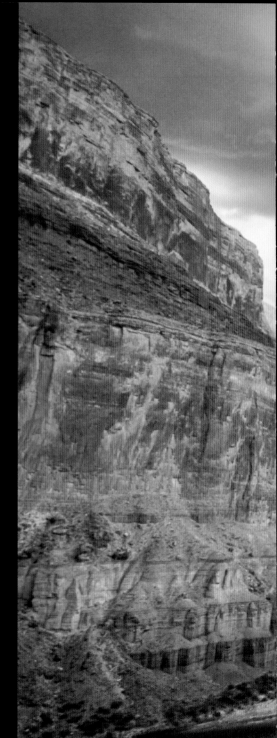

Above: This detail of a pictograph panel on a rock wall suggests the lives and mysteries of earlier people and animals in the Grand Canyon wilderness.

Right: Ancestral Puebloan ruins are sheltered within a shady rock alcove above the Colorado River at Nankoweap.

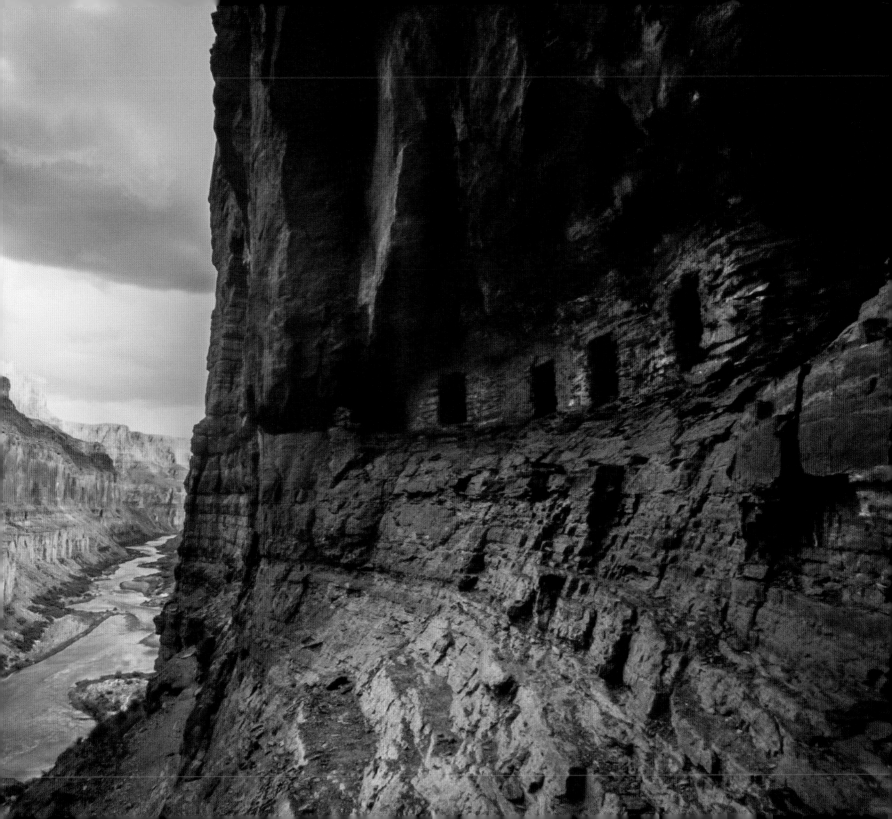

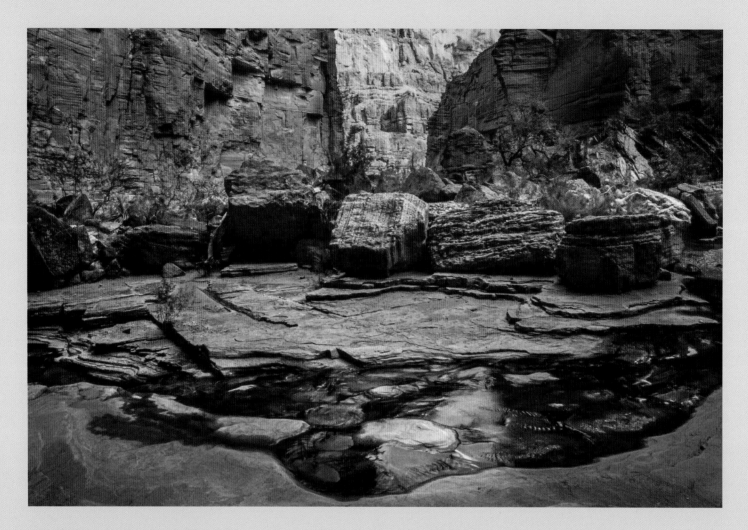

Above: Hiking up from the river into Matkatamiba Canyon, I found this composition of horizontal and vertical rock and the curve of a cool stream.

Facing page: Downstream from Upset Rapid, we rested briefly. I climbed up to capture the river canyon in a series of walled gates we had just passed through.

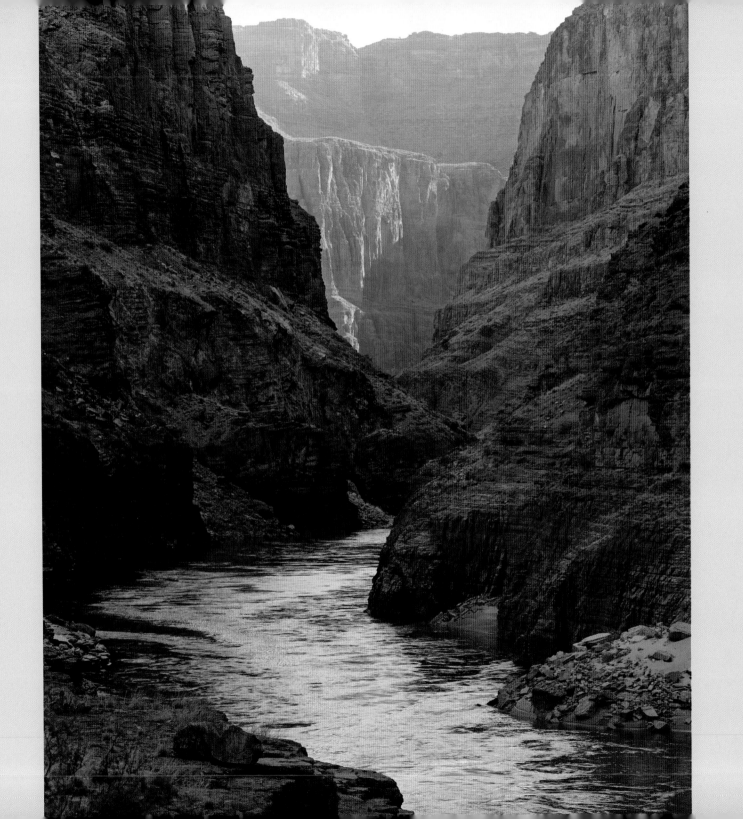

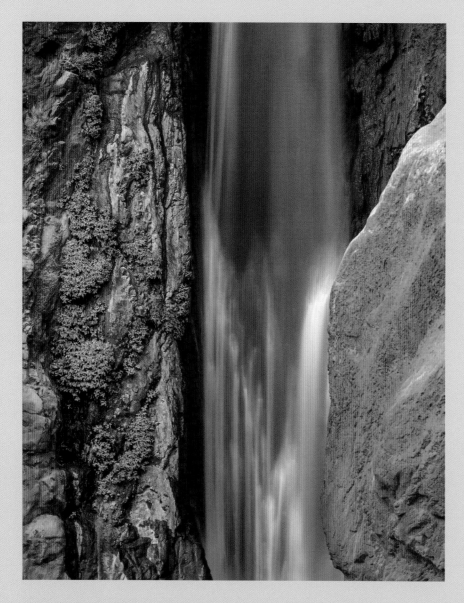

Above: I used a telephoto lens to make this image of Deer Creek Falls from river level.

Right: Clear Creek Falls off the North Kaibab Trail offers tantalizing shapes and designs of water cascading through the rock.

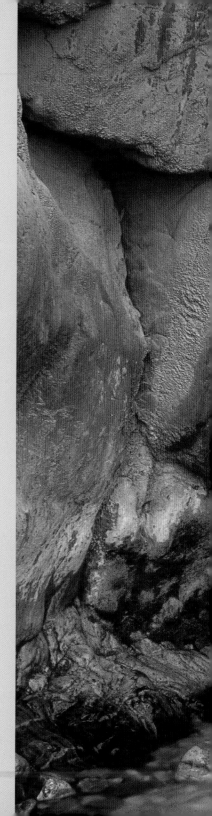

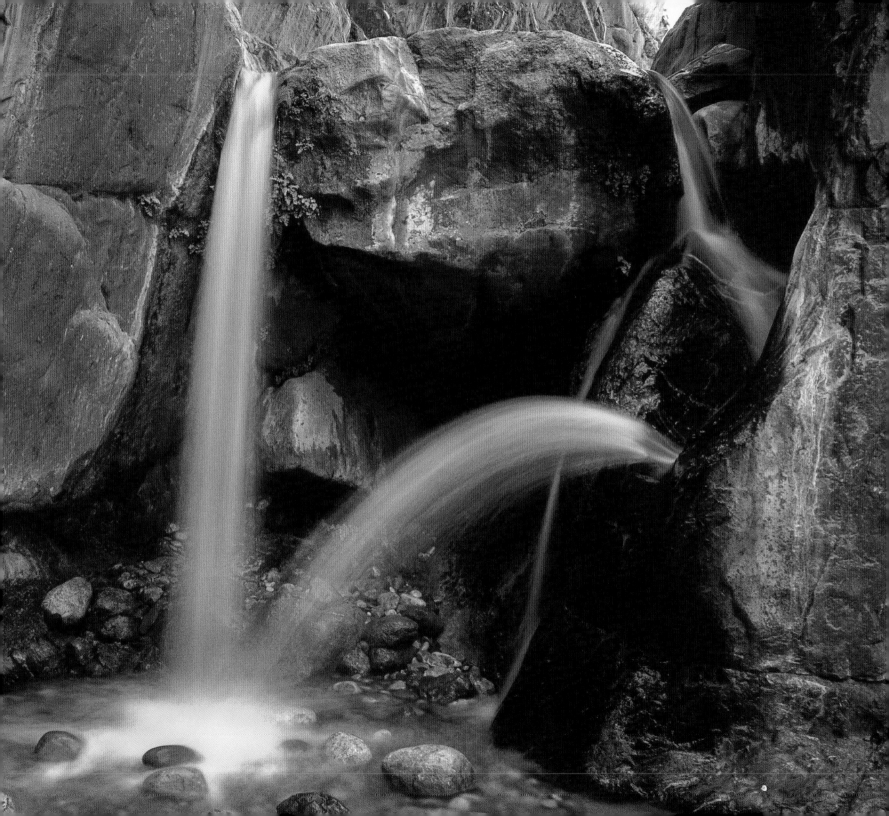

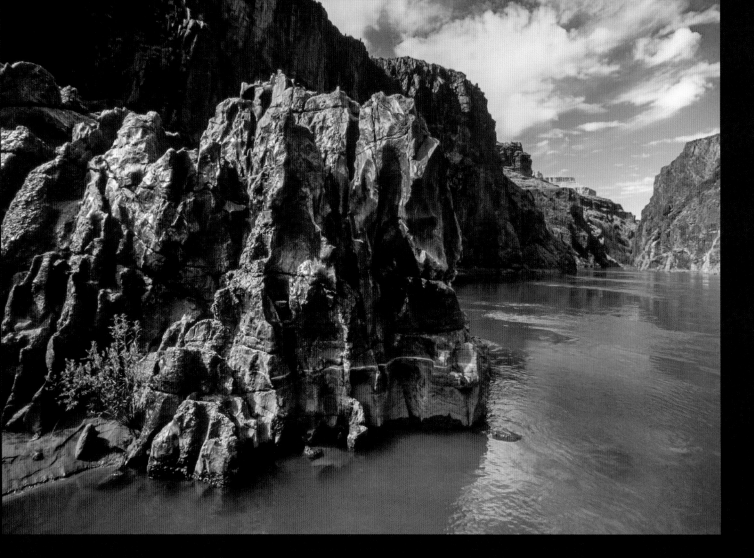

Above: Convoluted schist, the oldest rock layer in the inner gorge, demonstrates the river's carving power.
I had to stay in the boat to make this handheld shot, but my boatman tried to hold it steady.

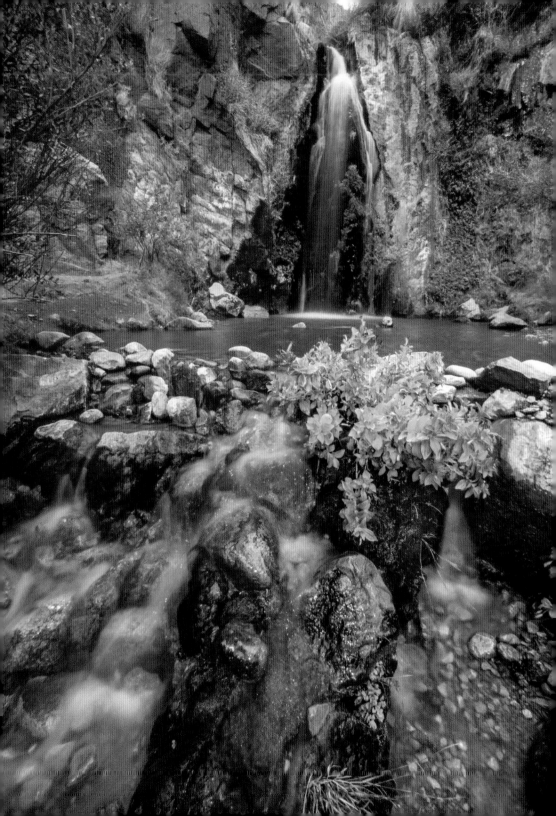

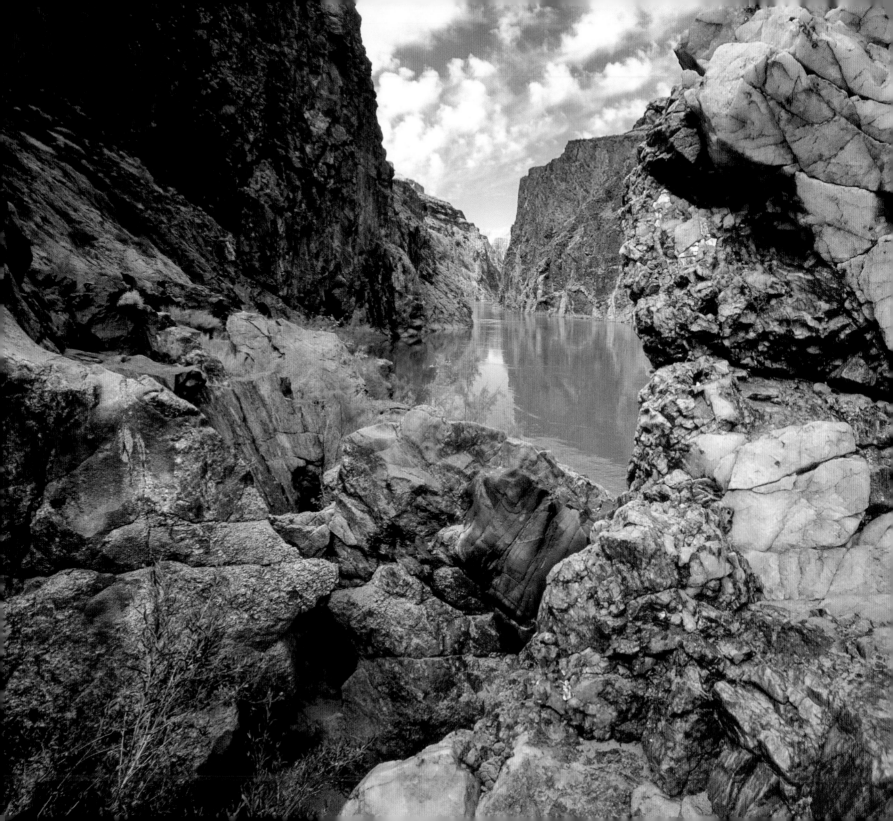

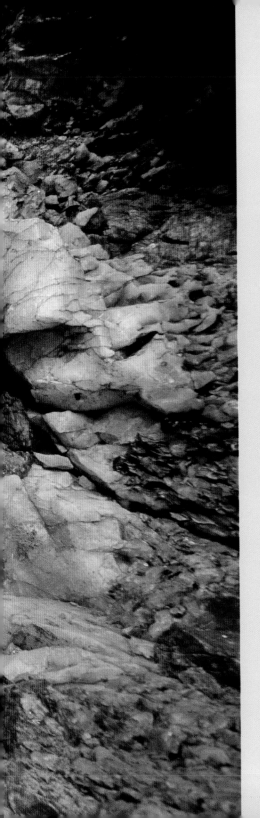

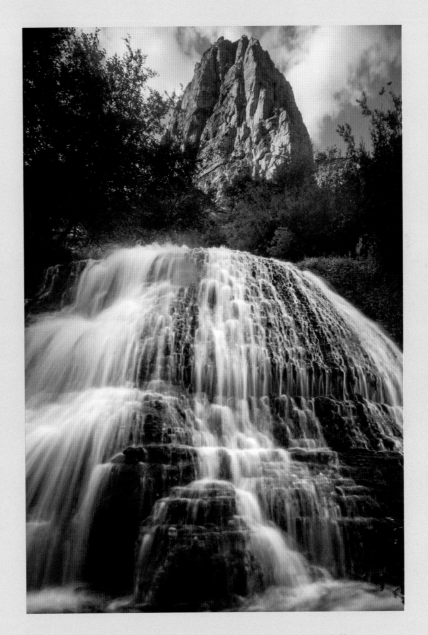

Above: Roaring Springs, along the Bright Angel Canyon trail below the North Rim, cascades to the Colorado River far below.

Left: My fascination with the details of conglomerate rock is an example of my natural connection with Lower Granite Gorge.

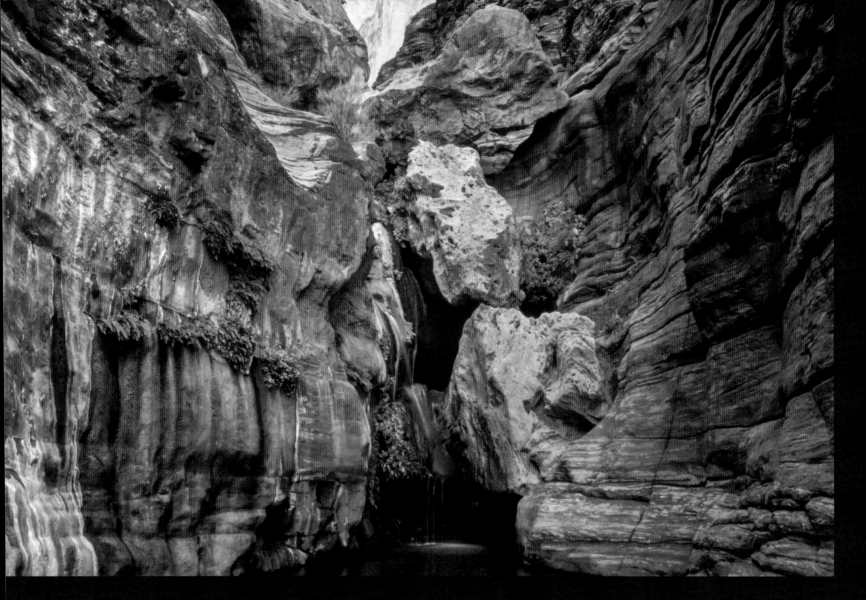

Above: Royal Arch Creek flows through Elves Chasm, a major stop on river trips. It is such a treat to hike up to this cool, shady oasis.

Facing page: Looking into Deer Creek Gorge on a hike up from the river, I can see how flash floods carve these magnificent side canyons.

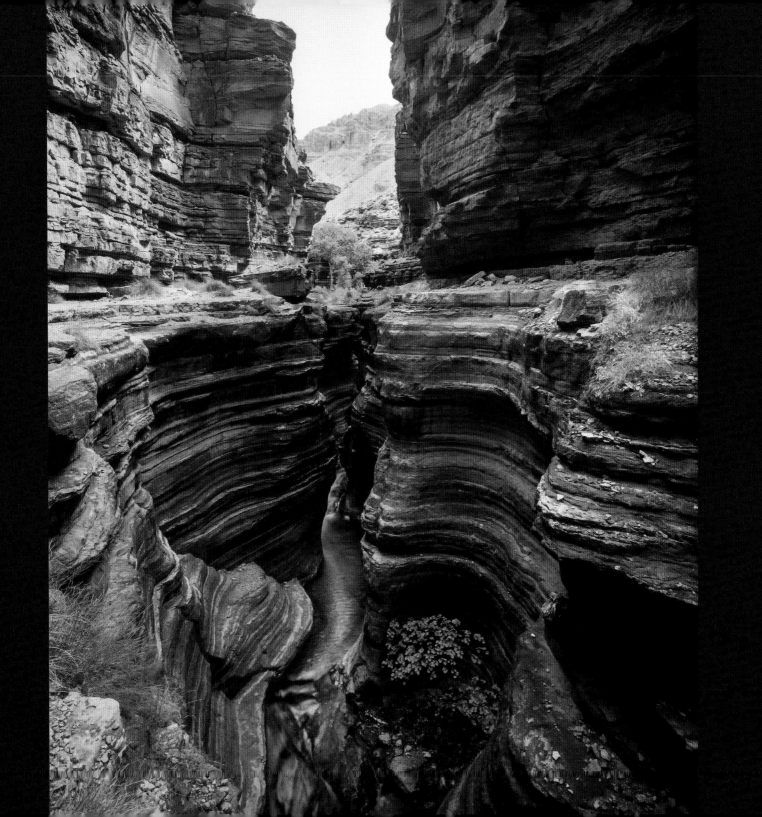

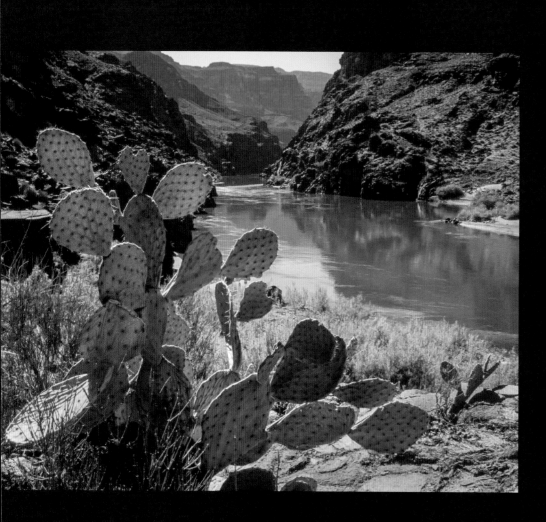

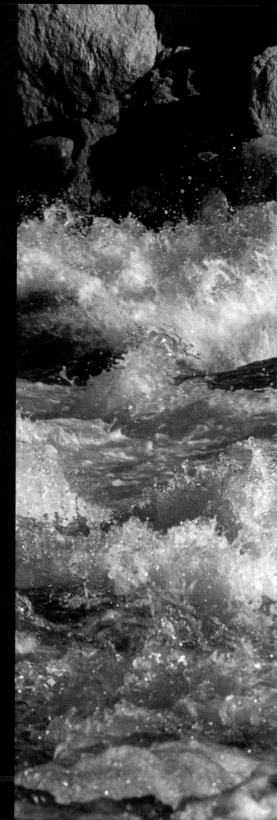

Above: Downstream from Upset Rapids, I took a short hike from the river rafts. I was intrigued by the contrast between the prickly pear cactus and greenery above the bank and the glassy section of river with a hint of the desert environment and rapids yet to come around the bends.

Right: I climbed out of the boat to make this image of Granite Rapids, then boulder-hopped among the rocks to catch up with my river companions after their exciting run. John Wesley Powell named this forbidding rapid on his exploration of the canyon in 1869. On river trips I kept my camera equipment in bags around my neck to protect it from water, mud, and dust. I needed both hands to hang on in whitewater, or scramble on the rocks.

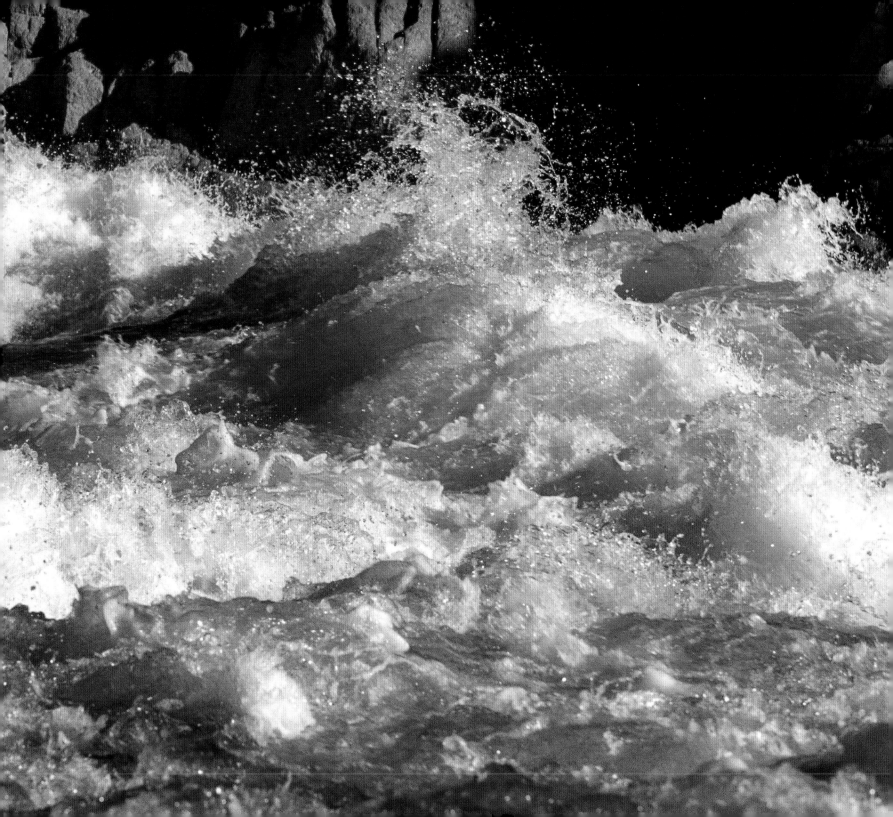

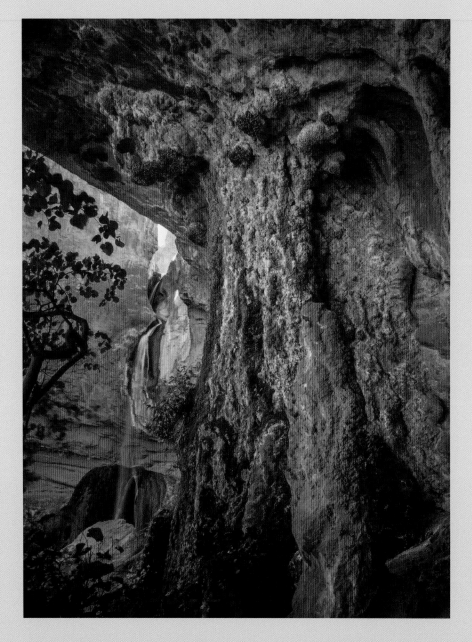

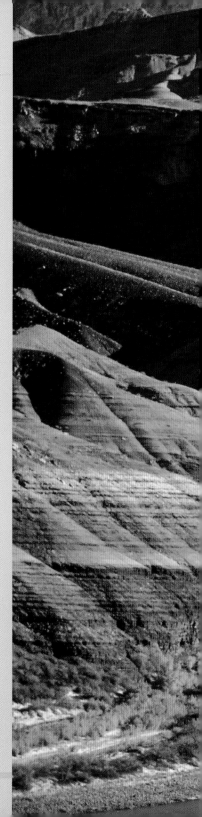

Above: From beneath an overhang of sandstone shapes, I made this image of Ribbon Falls in Bright Angel Canyon.

Right: The canyon heat is intense at Furnace Flats, where the river is flat and open. At our midday lunch stop, I hiked to a vantage above the water to record the placid curves of the Colorado River.

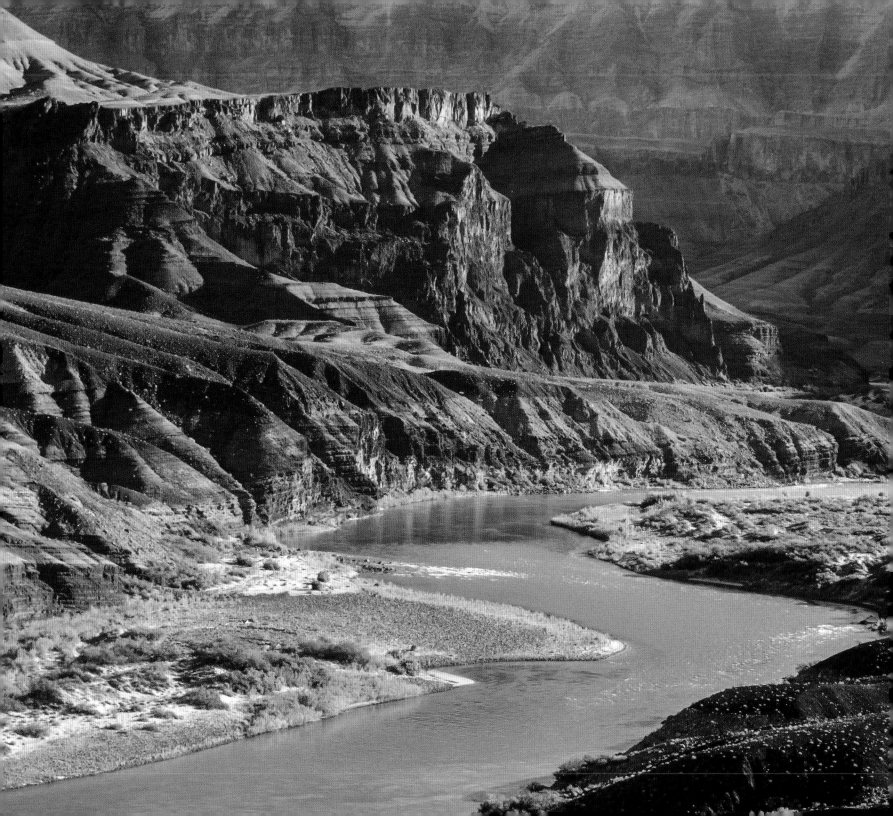

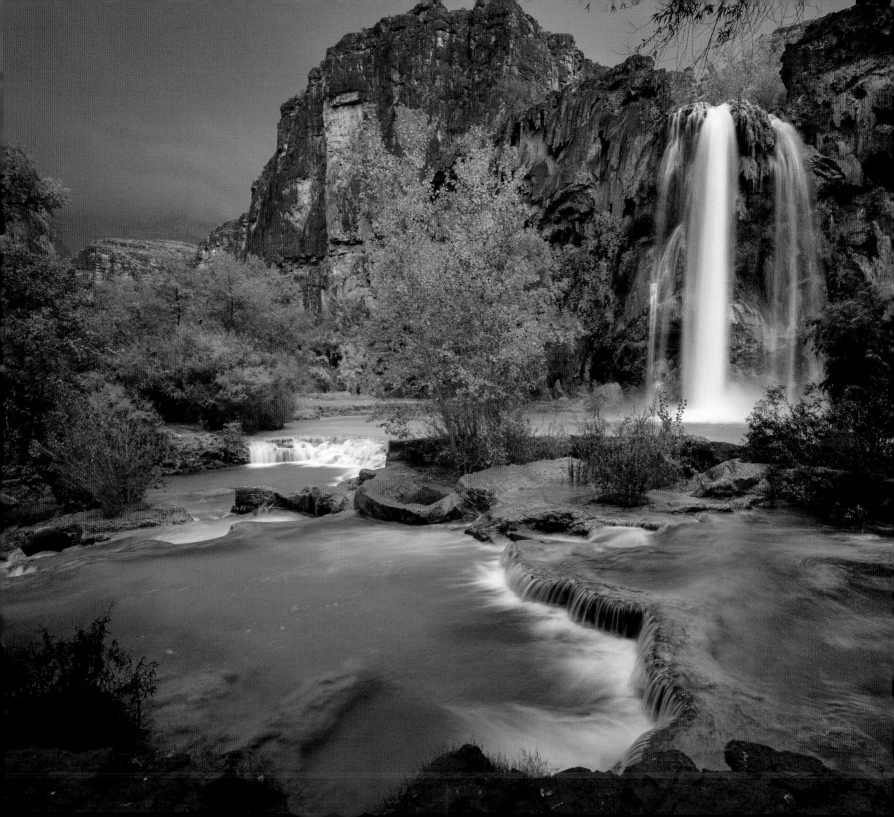

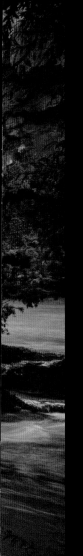

Left: On an autumn day, cloudy weather added drama as I made this image of Havasu Falls, on Havasupai tribal lands in the Grand Canyon.

Below: I hiked up from the river to reach these arresting blue-green travertine pools on Havasu Creek.

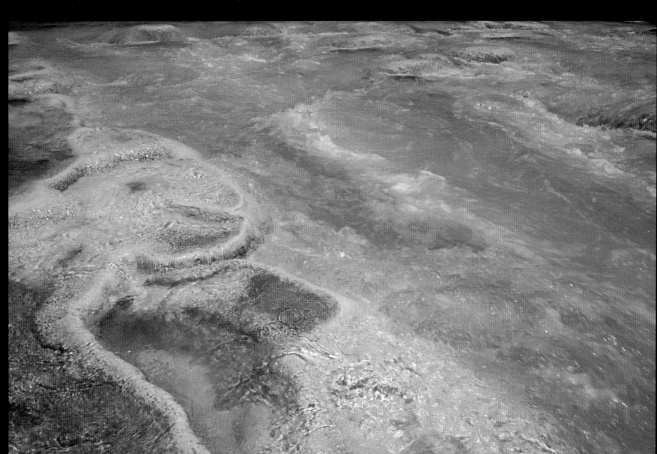

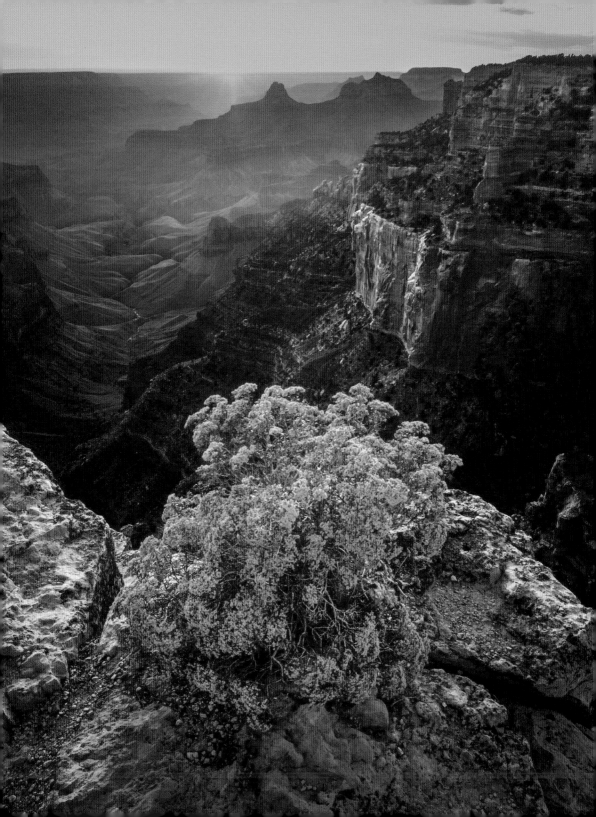

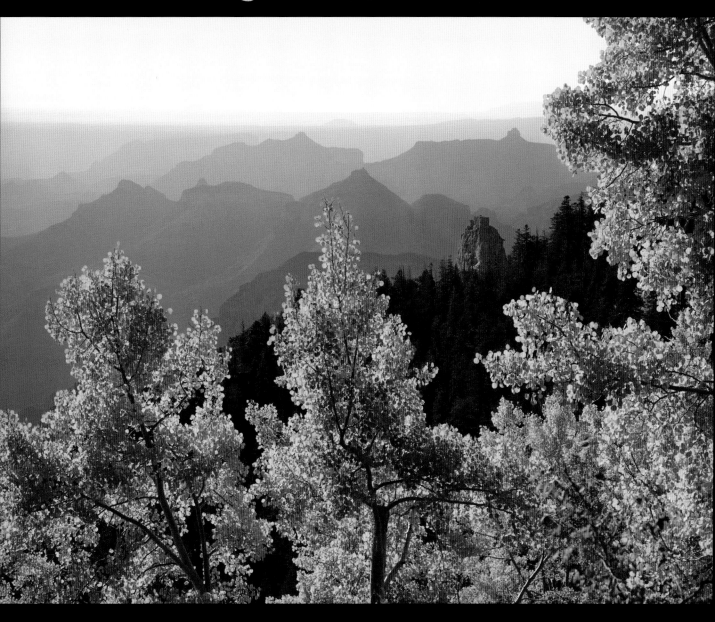

Above: Autumn-colored aspens frame an early morning view of Mount Hayden from Point Imperial.

Facing page: From the west side of Cape Royal, Zoroaster and Brahma Temples silhouette against the sunset.

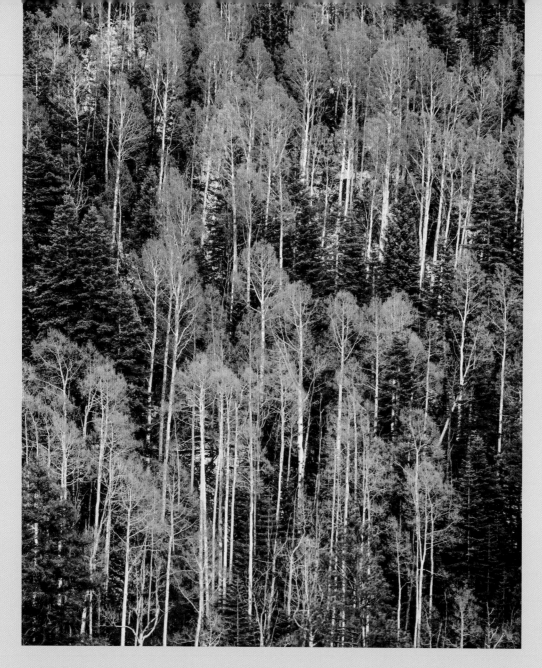

Above: An aspen grove in spring blends with dark green conifers on a hillside on the Grand Canyon's North Rim.

Right: On the North Rim between Cape Final and Cape Royal, I looked northeast past a ponderosa pine to views of Marble Canyon and the Vermillion Cliffs in the distance. I searched hard to locate this opening in the dense forest.

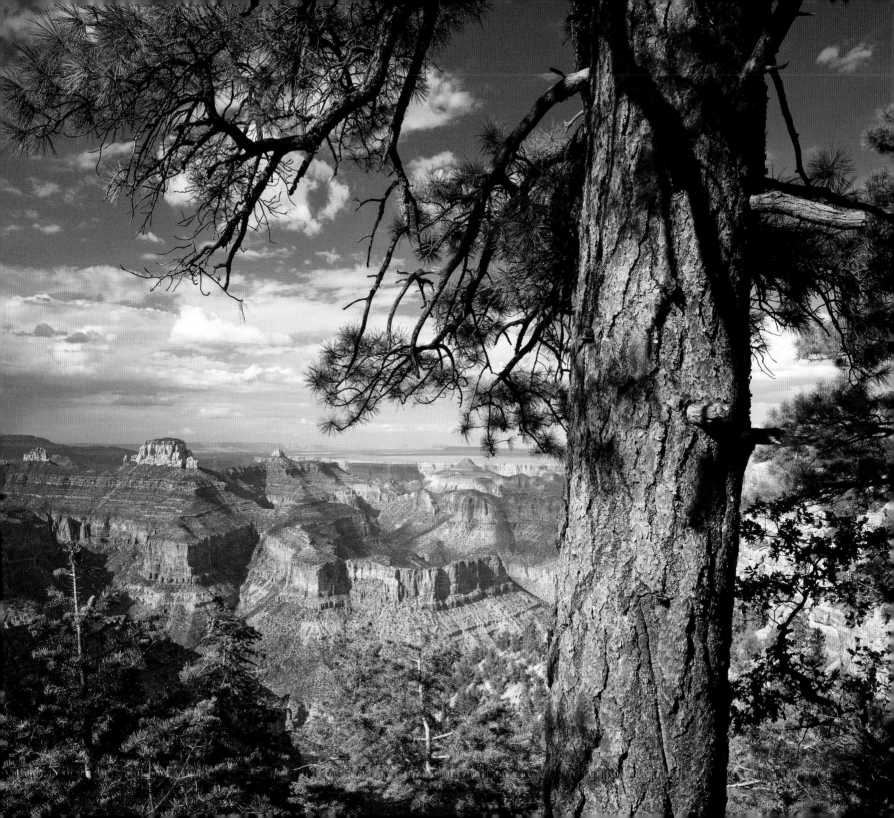

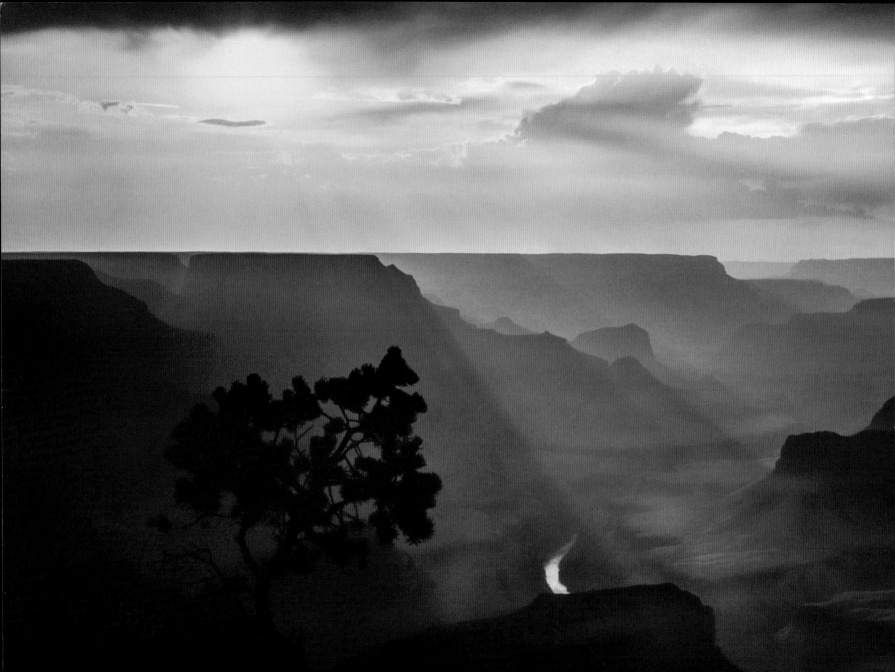

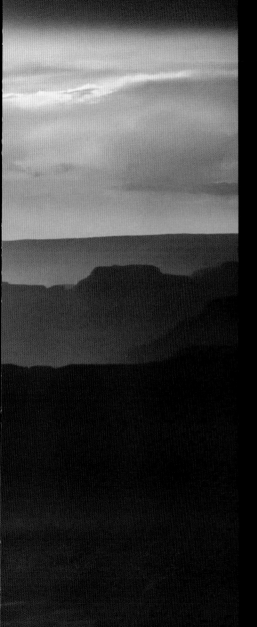

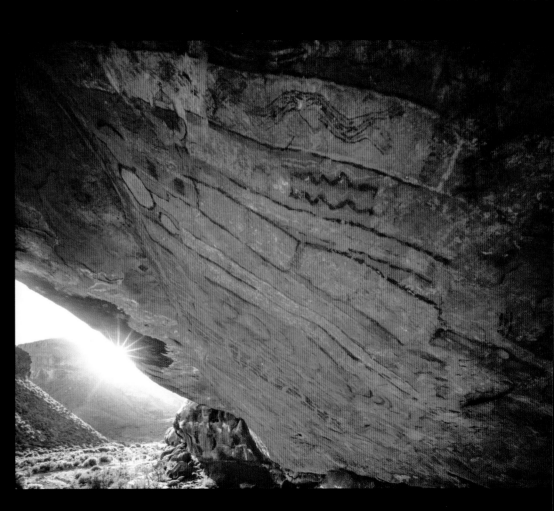

Above: A kiss of light beneath an overhead panel of pictographs required balance
between contrasting light densities.

Left: Evening light accents a stretch of the Colorado River deep in the Grand Canyon.

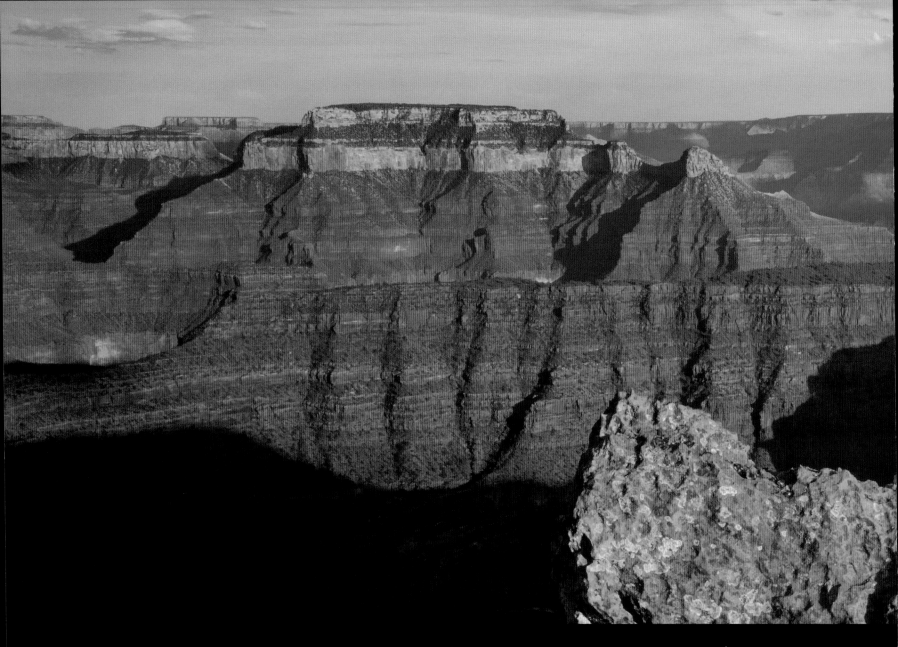

A wide panorama from Point Sublime encompasses Shiva, Menacious, and Confucious Temples, and late afternoon light on the rimrock.

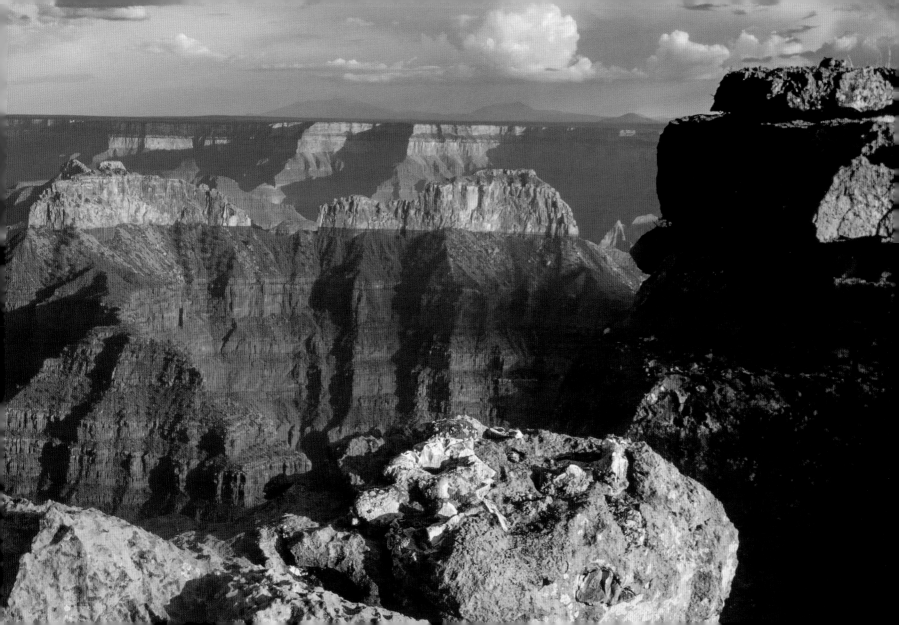

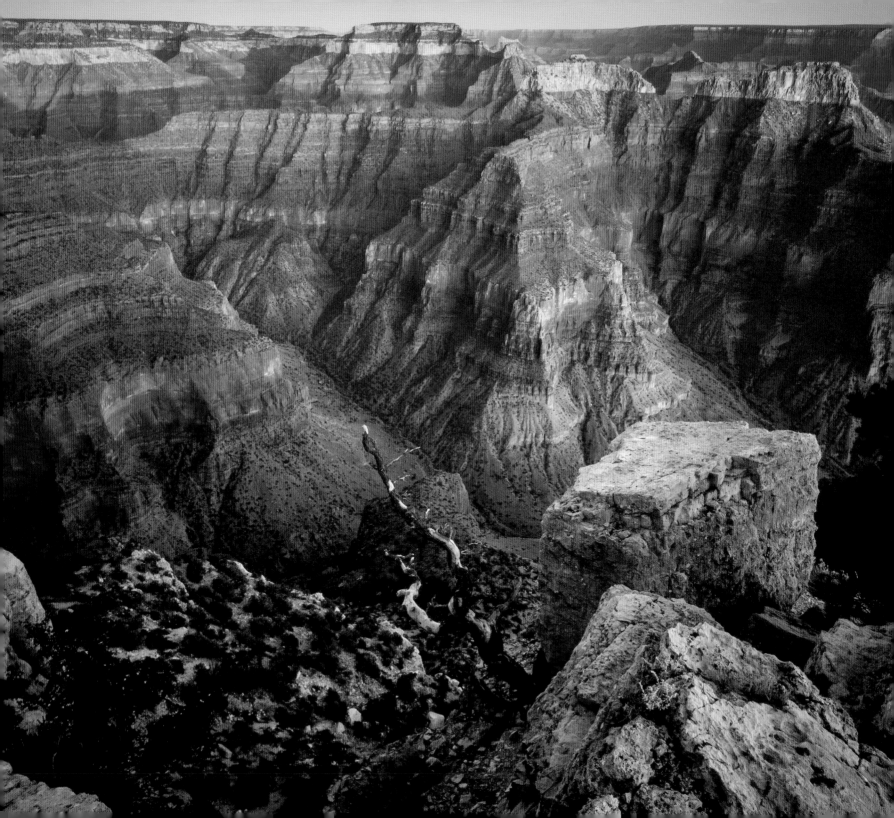

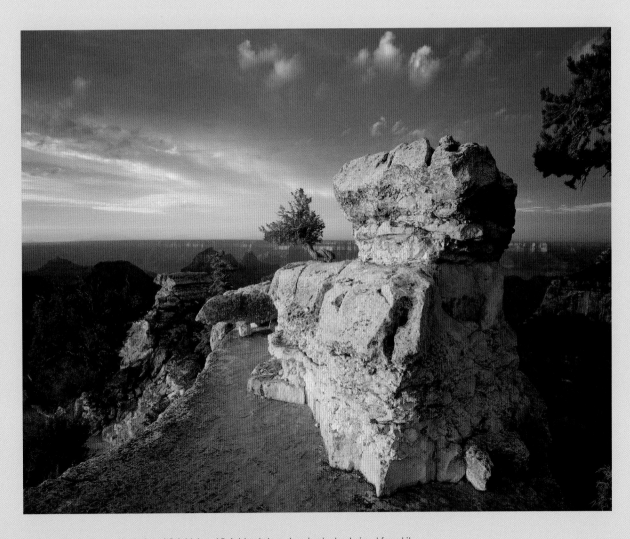

Above: The trail near the lodge at Bright Angel Point leads to a stunning lookout view. I found it enticing at sunrise with the distinctive rock feature in the foreground.

Left: I made this image from Point Sublime in the evening. Last light on the rims and a branch in the foreground emphasizes mysterious depths in the canyon.

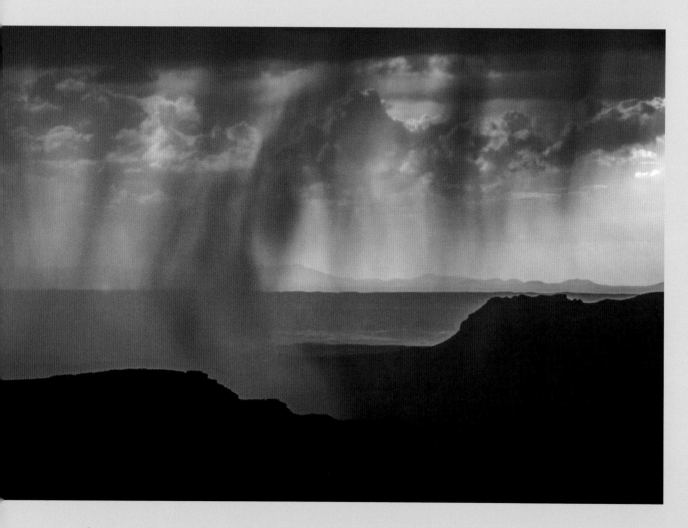

Above: Looking west from Point Sublime through a rain curtain, I saw the promise of changing light and weather in the clouds.

Right: Fast-changing light during a summer rainstorm suddenly lit Mount Hayden, viewed here from Point Imperial.

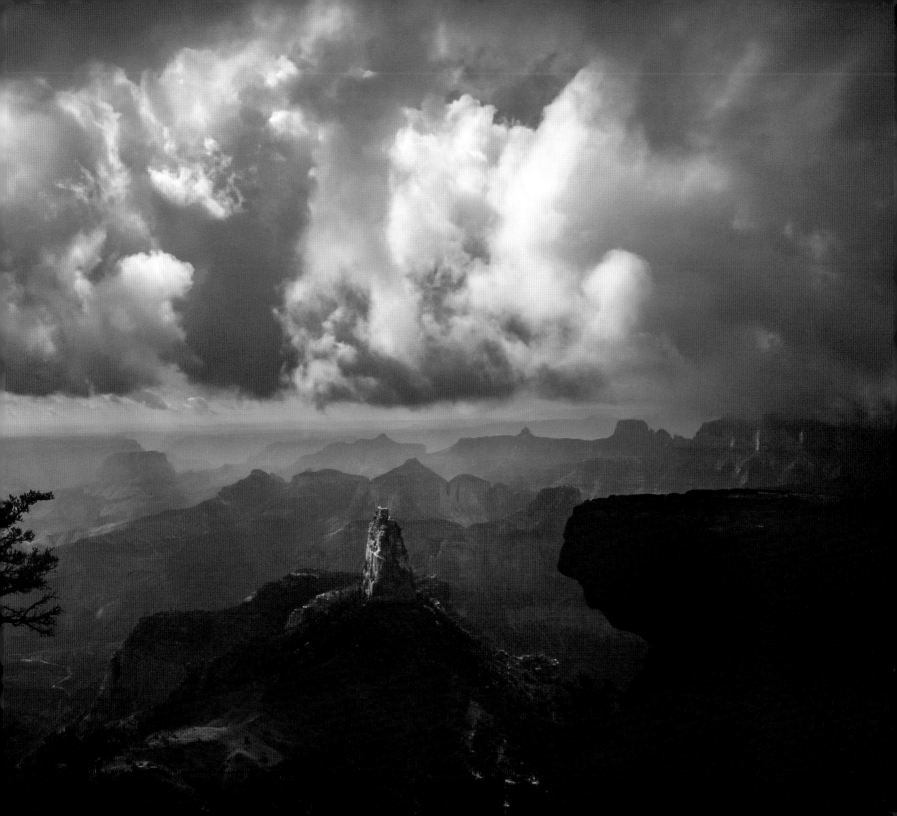

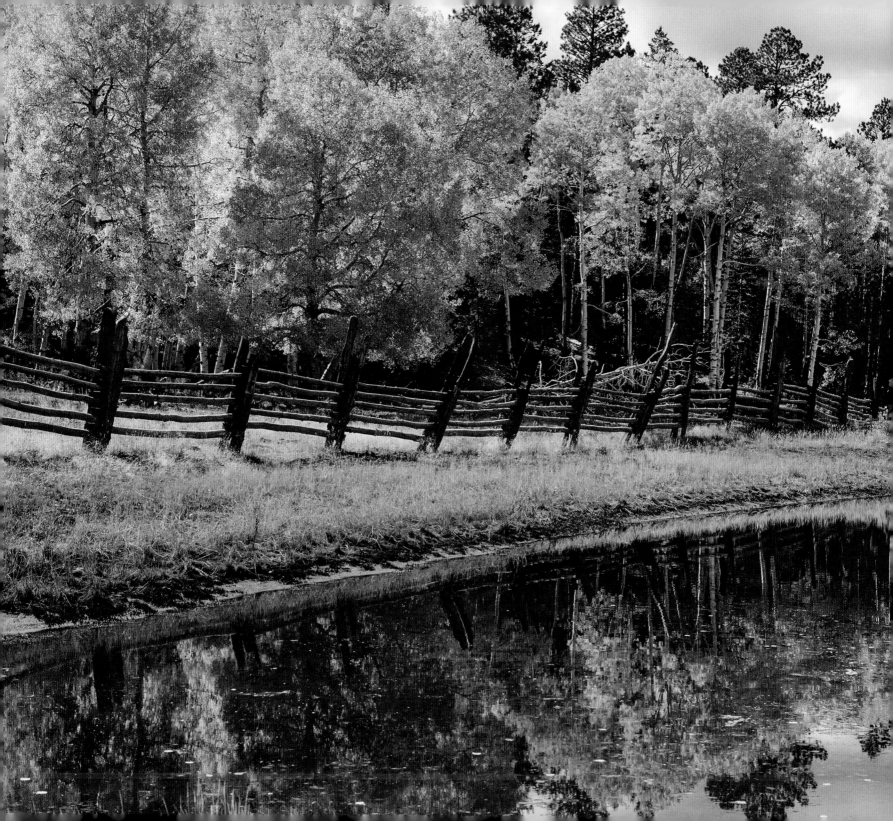

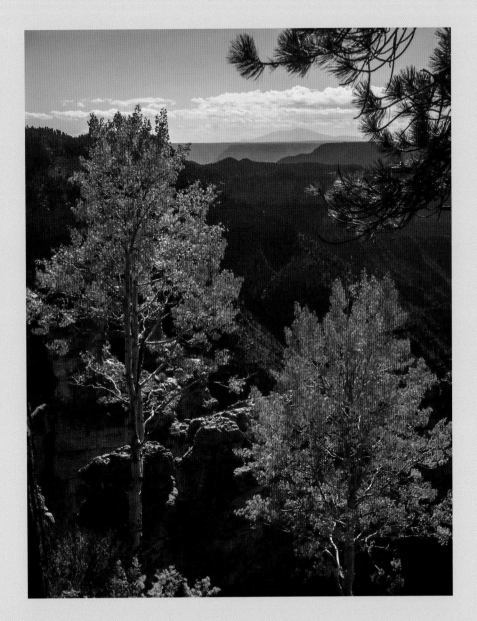

Above: Vivid color on the aspens is my celebration of a crisp autumn day on the North Rim. When snow falls, the North Rim roads will close until late spring.

Left: Fall color on the Kaibab Plateau gave me an opportunity to play with the reflection of trees, fence, and sky.

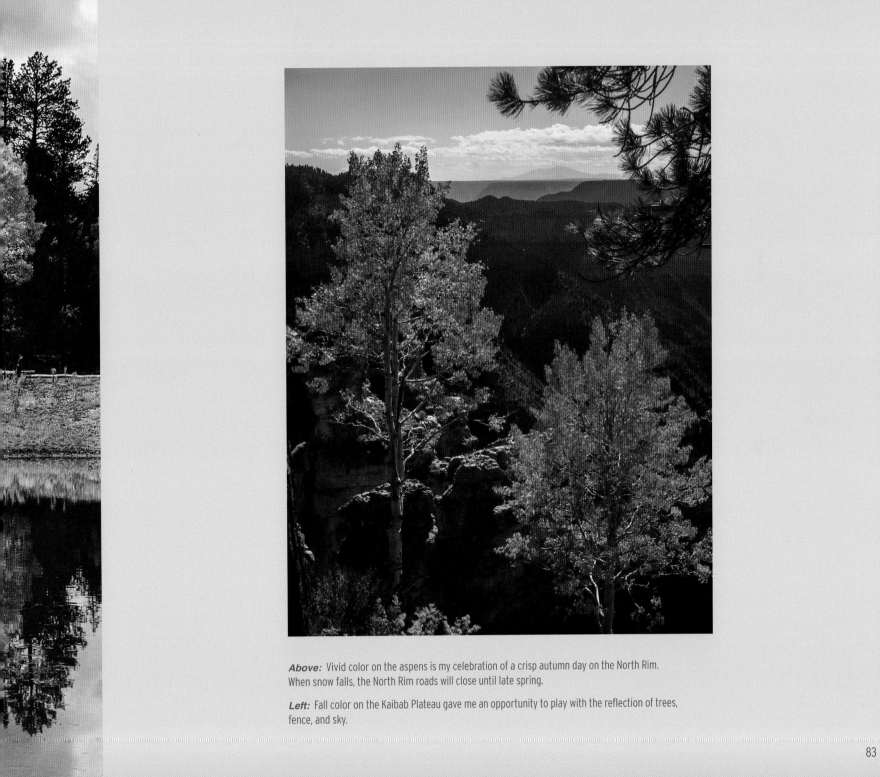

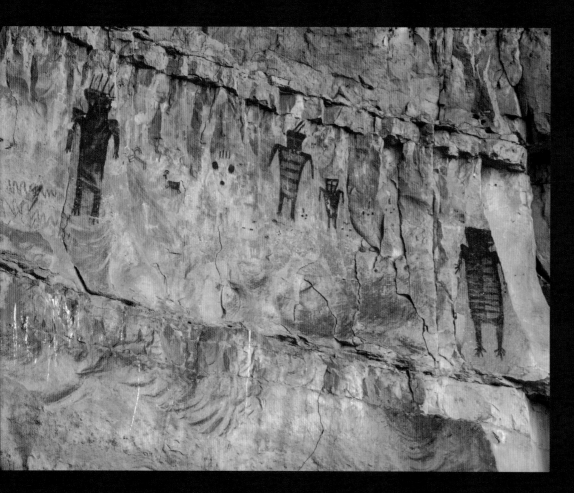

Above: I used a telephoto lens from below to shoot this pictograph panel.

Right: Late summer evening light casts a warm glow on Wotans Throne
and the buckwheat in bloom at my feet on the rimrock at Cape Royal.

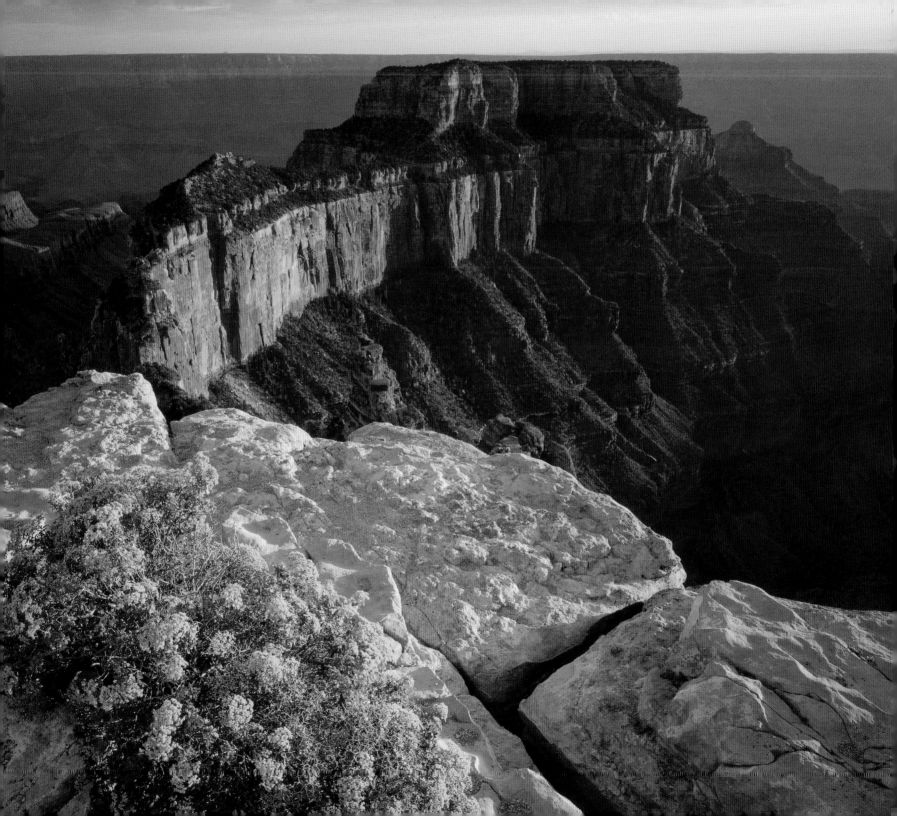

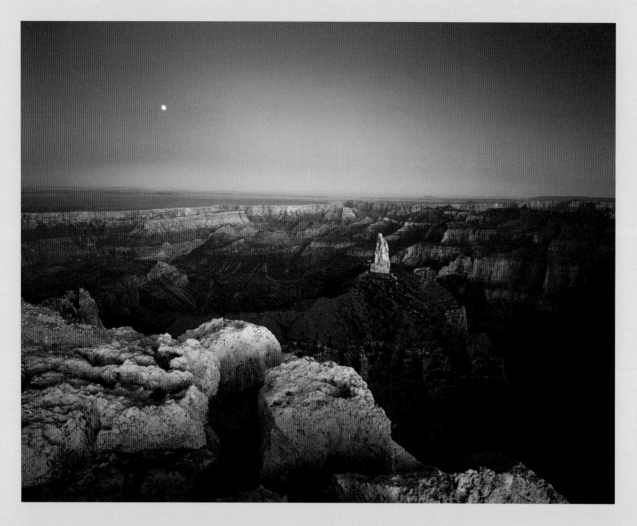

Above: From Point Imperial, I watched the moon rise as last light caught the pinnacle of Mount Hayden. The dark line below the sunset color is the earth's shadow.

Right: One evening at Toroweap West, the sunset colors streaked overhead. Lava Falls is visible on the Colorado River far below.

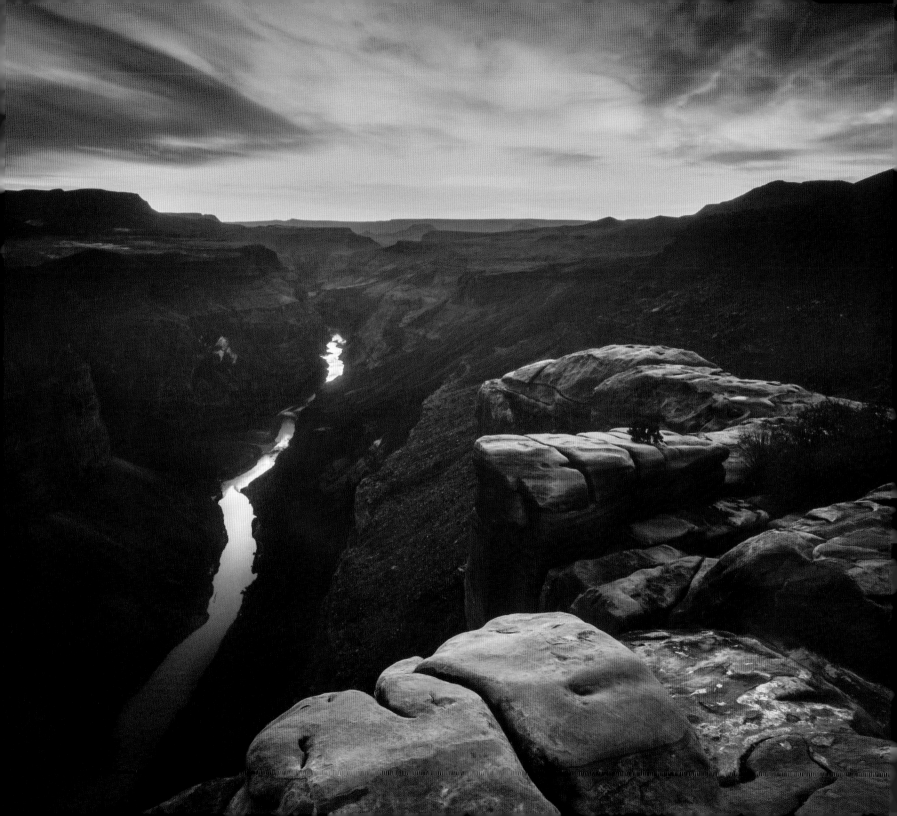

The Timeless Moment

My formal training at Rochester Institute of Technology in New York and Art Center College of Design in Los Angeles gave me mastery of the equipment, and prepared me for advertising agency assignment work. My "freestyle" work, the work of my heart, however, remained landscape. The painter Thomas Moran—who so wonderfully portrayed the stories of the large landscapes, the storms, the hanging clouds, the timescale of the landforms that became our national parks—strongly influenced me. My father, too, approached landscape photography in that dramatic, historical way. He taught me to shoot prolifically and thoroughly as I worked. I was also inspired by the great photography masters: Henri Cartier-Bresson, who addressed the "decisive moment"

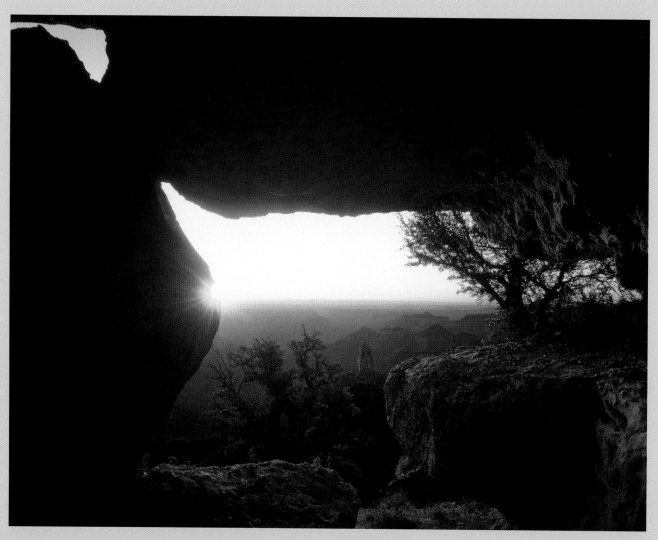

of an image as it tells the larger story, and Ernst Hass, whose spontaneous shooting with a handheld 35mm portrayed such expressive images in color. How, I wondered, could I "go painterly" like Moran and bring in the immediacy and emotion of Cartier-Bresson and Hass? The quest to make this happen sent me out into the landscape with unbounded passion.

After my schooling I delved into the fine-art thinking process and the challenge to make quintessential images worthy of exhibition prints. Edward Weston and Ansel Adams had established a high bar for black-and-white photographs of inspiring landscapes and still life. Their dedication to composition was a major influence on me.

Fascinated by the different qualities various film brings to a landscape image, I have made both black-and-white and color photos throughout my career—often of the same scene. The monochrome image might emphasize shapes more interestingly to me, or tell the viewer more about the subject, than a complex color one. I began to search for simplicity in composition, to let the story of the subject emerge. Brett Weston pushed the medium of art photography up to the edge of the abstract expressionist painters, his gelatin silver prints showing compelling ways to emphasize negative space. I found his work thrilling, especially the stark landscapes and

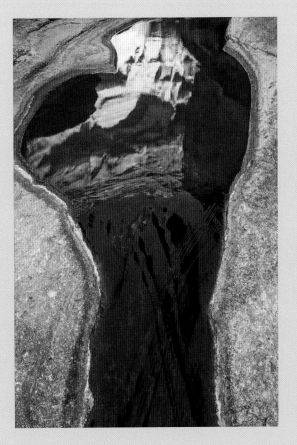

Above: A reflection pool captured my imagination on a river trip hike up Matkataniba Canyon.

Facing page: At the timeless moment of sunrise, I photographed Mount Hayden through a limestone window from Point Imperial on the North Rim.

pattern details. Ansel Adams' landscapes changed the character of nature photography in profound ways. We met early in my career in Yosemite National Park. He attended a show I had at Daniels Gallery in Carmel and invited me to visit him at his light-filled Carmel Highlands home, where he was very encouraging to me. Complimenting my work, Adams told me he had a lot of respect for my originality. These great photographers who inspired me were all masters of the "timeless moment." Their work remains inspiring and timeless to me today.

My own career in photography coincided with a rising need for editorial and advertising images, and the passion I had followed in exploring nature for myself developed into a successful career. I traveled widely, climbed peaks, descended canyons, and traversed the great landscapes of our planet with my cameras. I continue to do that. But seeing wilderness through my lens remained, and remains, the most exciting motive for me personally. I wanted to share the wildness I saw, to present the sense of the place through a photograph. Wanting to get past the "nice postcard" pictures taken in midday with lots of fluffy clouds, I yearned to find the most primal images—dramatic lighting, abstraction, and the coming and going edges of moody storms. I wanted to capture the mood and change I felt in each incredible wild location. In the early 1960s, my vision was very different from the norm.

In pursuit of the making of great photographs, I spent much of my career carrying a large 4x5 camera, setting up shots, and loading film, so the timing of these moments had to be exactly right. No matter how fast I could reload film, the next image wouldn't be what the first was. Now, with digital photography, I can be much more immediate. I sketch with my camera, exploring the limits of my equipment, to expand my creativity. I have the freedom to explore more possibilities with every subject. Still, each moment has its own emotion, its own time. Every time I return to my favorite places and subjects—like the Grand Canyon—I try new images, with new passion and vision. I try new vantage points, or different approaches, to show the viewer my natural connection to the place. I want to show my emotions at the moment the image was captured. ❖

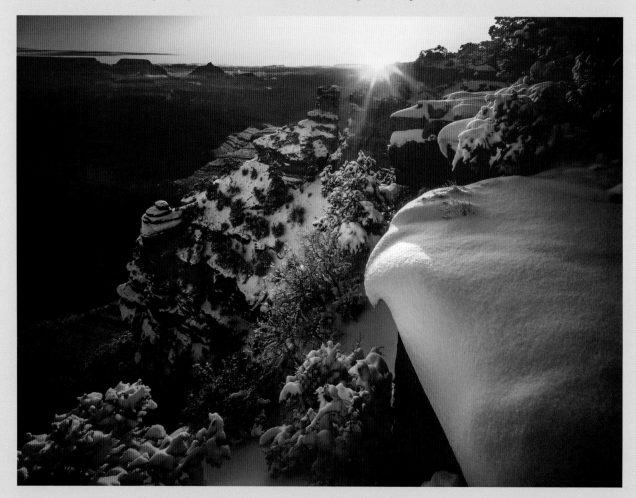

Right: On the South Rim near Powell Point, the rising sun highlights a hook of snow-covered rock.

Facing page: At sunrise, winter morning fog offers magical light near Mather Point.

Photographing the Grand Canyon

I study the seasons, the weather systems, the shadows, and the light when I visit Grand Canyon National Park. In summer, the monsoon season, I might see massive clouds build and a thunderstorm break open. I might get wet…what could be better than that? A scene that was ordinary in my lens in the late morning might be incredible in the late afternoon. A rising fog or an overcast day might give me the opportunity for a more dramatic image. I like to work with backlight, and now with the digital process I can remove flares, so I am freer to be creative and make many more images than I did with film. At the Grand Canyon, winter's short days offer incredible opportunities for detail and contrasts. Snow in this usually arid world brings a special dimension and a different emotional weight to my images. After a summer rain, a reflection in a rain pool might be a very intimate, personal way to express how I felt when the shadows and weather changed.

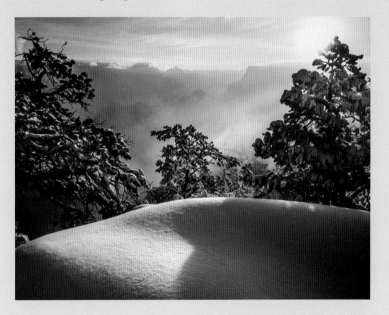

I look for the feeling of "near-far" in a landscape with a big sky. I move around and let the sky give me space—the exceptionally wide space the Grand Canyon is known for. How can I make an image of a huge vista more intimate, more personal? What if instead of standing on a rock to get the widest vista, I used that rock in my foreground? Is there an element in the near—a cactus flower or weathered wood snag—that will help make the rock forms marching into the distance even more dramatic?

Side light, rather than harsh bright light, can help me capture more subtle forms. Interesting textures develop when working in low-contrast, softer light. I follow patterns in the scene right before me. I look for repeating lines, diagonal formations, and even vertical compositions in this very horizontal country. Lines of color—autumn trees against red rock or blue shadows—might lead me to discover an interesting hidden part of a scene. Then…I wait. I slow down, breathe in, and let myself see the full range of what is before me, from just beneath my feet to the widest vista.

Sometimes, it's simply so beautiful in the moment that a photographer just needs to capture the shot. If the landscape in every direction is incredible, I make plenty of images—no need to be over-technical. When I review and edit my images later, I keep those that best represent my most compelling natural connections to the Grand Canyon experience.

I seek to express my sense of place as I capture the mood of a scene. Will my image show how I felt, how the layers of rock and time moved me? Will it be a "timeless moment" between past and future? Does the near foreground help place me in the larger world of the immense background? I don't just take a picture—through my work, I strive to make an image meaningful to myself and to those who will view the ever-changing and infinite grandeur of this place of eternity. ❖

About the Images

The photographs in this book span five decades. Most of the images were shot as 4x5, large format, Kodak Ektachrome and Fuji Velvia color film. My primary camera in my early years of photography was a Linhof Technika, usually on a tripod. I later worked with a Leicaflex and Canon. In recent years,

I've been enjoying the spontaneity of digital photography using a Panasonic Lumix.

See more of my American landscape and nature photography, particularly Portfolio #16 for more images of Grand Canyon National Park, at www.davidmuenchphotography.com. ❖

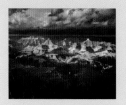

Front cover and page 35: Winter, near Yavapai Point. Linhof 4x5, 75mm lens. 1966.

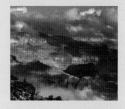

Title page: Morning Mood, South Rim. Linhof 4x5, 210mm lens. 1966.

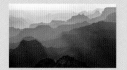

Page 2-3: Canyon Ridges from Desert View. Linhof 4x5, 300mm telephoto lens. 1994.

Page 5: Moonrise, Yaki Point. Linhof 4x5, 500mm telephoto lens. 1995.

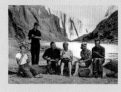

Page 6: Glen Canyon. Photo by Josef Muench, c. 1955.

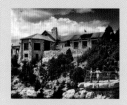

Page 7: North Rim Lodge. Photo by Josef Muench, c. 1950.

Page 8: *Top:* photo by Josef Muench, c. 1946. *Bottom:* Marc Muench at South Rim. 35mm. 1976.

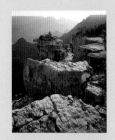

Page 9: Rimrock, Mather Point. Linhof 4x5, 75mm lens. 1992.

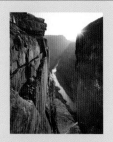

Page 10: Toroweap Sunrise. Linhof 4x5, 75mm wide angle lens. 1970.

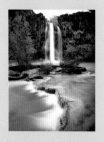

Page 11: Havasu Falls. Linhof 4x5, 75mm lens. 2003.

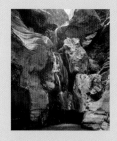

Page 12: Elves Chasm. Linhof 4x5, 90mm lens. 1966.

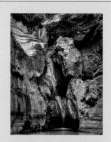

Page 13: Elves Chasm Revisited. Linhof 4x5, 90mm lens. 1998.

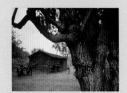

Page 15: Historic Cabin, Lees Ferry. Linhof 4x5, 75mm lens. 1995.

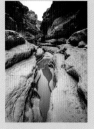

Page 16: Cathedral Canyon. Linhof 4x5, 75mm wide angle lens. 1995.

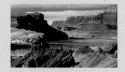

Page 17: Lees Ferry. Linhof 4x5, 90mm lens. 1995.

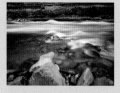

Page 18: Rapid in Marble Canyon. Linhof 4x5, 210mm lens; slow exposure 30 seconds. 1995.

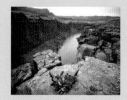

Page 19: Beavertail Cactus. Linhof 4x5, 75mm wide angle lens. 1985.

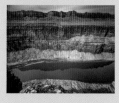

Page 20: Colorado River, Marble Canyon. Linhof 4x5, 75mm wide angle lens. 1997.

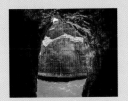

Page 21: Rock Window, Marble Canyon. 21mm Leicaflex. 1997.

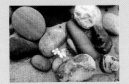

Page 22: Primrose and River Cobbles. 35mm Leicaflex, 50mm lens. 1995.

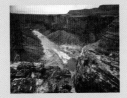

Page 23: Badger Rapids. Linhof 4x5, 90mm lens. 1995.

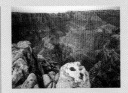

Page 24: Dawn above the Confluence. Linhof 4x5, 90mm lens. 1995.

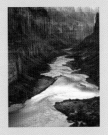

Page 25: Colorado River at Nankoweap. 35mm Leicaflex, 90mm lens. 1975.

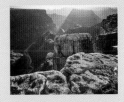

Page 26: Above the Confluence. Linhof 4x5, 75mm wide angle lens. 1997.

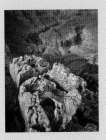

Page 27: Tatahatso Point. Linhof 4x5, 75mm wide angle lens. 1997.

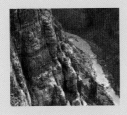

Page 28: Little Colorado River. Linhof 4x5, 300mm lens. 1997.

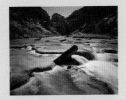

Page 29: Little Colorado Terraces. Linhof 4x5, 75mm lens. 1997.

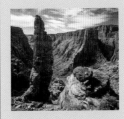

Page 30: Sandstone Pinnacle. Linhof 4x5, 90mm lens. 1997.

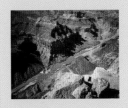

Page 31: Comanche Point. Linhof 4x5, 75mm lens. 1997.

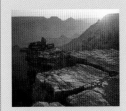

Page 32: Rimrock Sunrise. Linhof 4x5, 75mm lens. 1994.

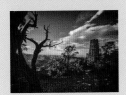

Page 33: Desert View Watchtower. 35mm Leicaflex, 21mm lens. 1975.

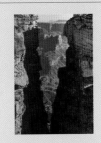

Page 34: Limestone Rim V-Cut. 35mm Leicaflex, 135mm telephoto lens. 1998.

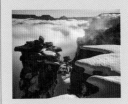

Page 36: Morning Fog, South Rim. Linhof 4x5, 90mm lens. 1969.

(Page 35: see front cover.)

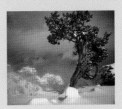

Page 37: Juniper and Clearing Storm. Linhof 4x5, 210mm lens. 1978.

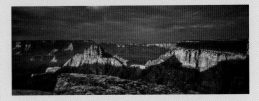

Pages 38-39: Coronado Butte. Linhof 4x5, 75mm lens panorama. 1994.

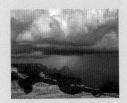

Page 40: Snowstorm near Navajo Point. Linhof 4x5, 90mm lens. 1975.

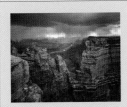

Page 41: Rain Curtain, Desert View. Linhof 4x5, 300mm telephoto lens. 1975.

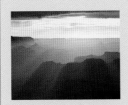

Page 42: Sunset Ridges, Lipan Point. Linhof 4x5, 210mm lens. 1997.

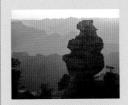

Page 43: Balanced Rock. Linhof 4x5, 300mm lens. 1970.

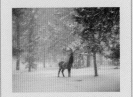

Page 44: Elk in Ponderosa Forest. 35mm Canon, 135mm lens. 2009.

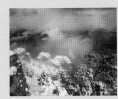

Page 45: Clearing Winter Storm. Linhof 4x5, 90mm lens. 1978.

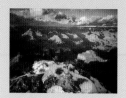

Page 46: Powell Point Winterscape. Linhof 4x5, 90mm lens. 1978.

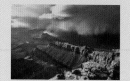

Page 47: Lipan Point Rainshower. 35mm Leicaflex, 90mm lens. 1975.

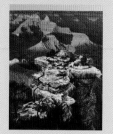

Page 48: Shadowed Rimrock, Yavapai Point. Linhof 4x5, 210mm lens. 1994.

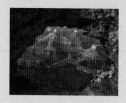

Page 49: Limestone Window. Linhof 4x5, 210mm lens. 1994.

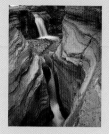

Page 50: Deer Creek Gorge. Linhof 4x5, 90mm lens. 1975.

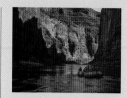

Page 51: Rafting Still Waters. 35mm Leicaflex, 90mm lens. 1975.

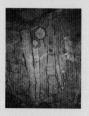

Page 52: Pictograph Panel. Linhof 4x5, 90mm lens, 1975.

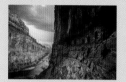

Page 53: Ruins at Nankoweap. 35mm Leicaflex, 21mm lens. 1975.

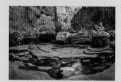

Page 54: Matkataniba Canyon. 35mm Leicaflex, 21mm lens. 1995.

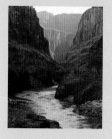

Page 55: Downstream from Upset Rapid. Linhof 4x5, 210mm lens, 1966.

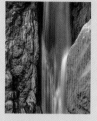

Page 56: Deer Creek Falls. Linhof 4x5, 300mm lens. 1967.

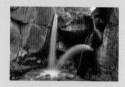

Page 57: Clear Creek Falls. 35mm Leicaflex, 90mm lens. 1967.

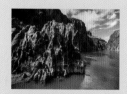

Page 58: Convoluted Schist, Inner Gorge. 35mm Leicaflex, 21mm lens. 1967.

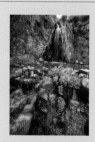

Page 59: Stone Creek Falls. 35mm Leicaflex, 21mm lens. 1966.

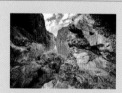

Page 60: Lower Granite Gorge. 35mm Leicaflex, 21mm lens. 1966.

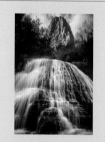

Page 61: Roaring Springs. Linhof 4x5, 90mm lens. 1970.

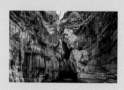

Page 62: Royal Arch Creek. 35mm Leicaflex, 21mm lens. 1995.

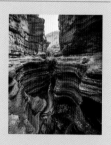

Page 63: Carved Walls, Deer Creek Gorge. Linhof 4x5, 75mm lens. 1966.

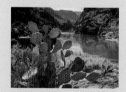

Page 64: Prickly Pear. 35mm Leicaflex, 21mm lens. 1995.

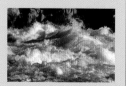

Page 65: Granite Rapids. 35mm Leicaflex, 135mm telephoto lens. 1995.

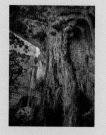

Page 66: Ribbon Falls. Linhof 4x5, 90mm lens. 1987.

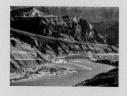

Page 67: Furnace Flats. Linhof 4x5, 210mm lens. 1966.

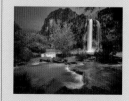

Page 68: Havasu Falls. Linhof 4x5, 75mm lens. 1999.

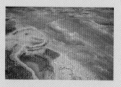

Page 69: Havasu Creek. 35mm Leicaflex, 90mm lens. 1999.

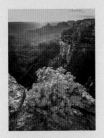

Page 70: Cape Royal. Linhof 4x5, 75mm wide angle lens. 1998.

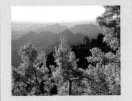

Page 71: Point Imperial, Autumn. Linhof 4x5, 90mm lens. 1966.

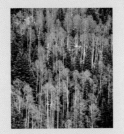

Page 72: Aspen Grove in Spring. Linhof 4x5, 500mm telephoto lens. 1997.

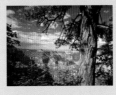

Page 73: Cape Final. Linhof 4x5, 75mm lens. 1997.

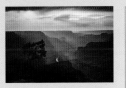

Page 74: Bright Angel Point Sunset. Linhof 4x5, 90mm lens. 1966.

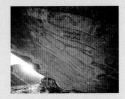

Page 75: Overhang with Pictographs. Linhof 4x5, 90mm lens. 1975.

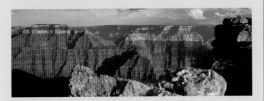

Pages 76-77: Temples from Point Sublime. Linhof 4x5, 75mm lens, cropped to panorama. 1994.

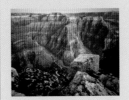

Page 78: Point Sublime Depths. Linhof 4x5, 75mm lens. 1994.

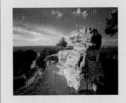

Page 79: Bright Angel Point. Linhof 4x5, 75mm lens. 1994.

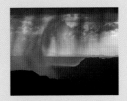

Page 80: Rain Curtain, North Rim. 35mm Leicaflex, 135mm lens. 1994.

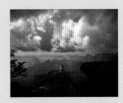

Page 81: Rainstorm, Mount Hayden. Linhof 4x5, 75mm lens. 1998.

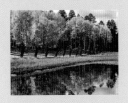

Page 82: Autumn Pond Reflection. Linhof 4x5, 90mm lens. 1985.

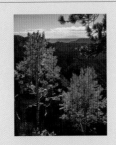

Page 83: Vivid Aspens, North Rim. Linhof 4x5, 90mm lens. 1994.

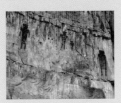

Page 84: Old Ones, Pictographs. Linhof 4x5, 300mm lens. 1975.

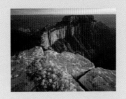

Page 85: Wotans Throne from Cape Royal. Linhof 4x5, 75mm lens. 1995.

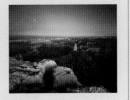

Page 86: Point Imperial Moonrise. Linhof 4x5, 75mm lens. 1995.

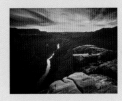

Page 87: Toroweap West Sunset. Linhof 4x5, 75mm lens. 1998.

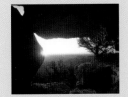

Page 88: Window, Point Imperial. Linhof 4x5, 90mm lens. 1995.

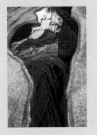

Page 89: Reflection Pool. 35mm Leicaflex, 90mm lens. 1966.

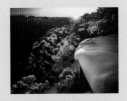

Page 90: Powell Point Sunrise. Linhof 4x5, 75mm lens. 1997.

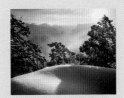

Page 91: Mather Point Sunrise. Linhof 4x5, 210mm lens. 1997.

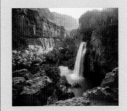

Page 96: Havasu Falls, Havasuapi Lands. Linhof 4x5, 75mm lens. 1985.s

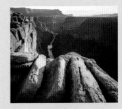

Back cover: Toroweap East. Linhof 4x5, 75mm lens. 1970.

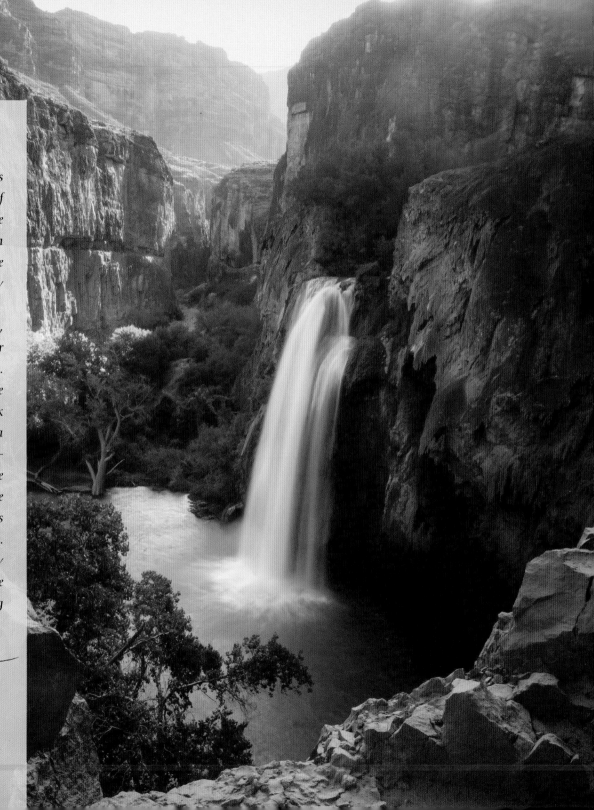

Acknowledgments

My inspiration for this book stretches back to my parents, Joyce and Josef Muench. My travels with them in the Grand Canyon introduced me to an intimacy with this place and with the natural landscape that formed my way of life.

I am grateful to my own children, Zandria and Marc, and to their mother Bonnie, for sharing my life's travels. I thank my personal assistant, Page Morgan, for the behind-the-scenes work that makes the accomplishment of a book possible, and my editorial consultant, Jane Freeburg at Collaborative Publishing Services, for connecting me with the great people at Farcountry Press and word-smithing this book to fruition.

And a very special thank you to my wife, Ruth, for her unending patience with me and for her love and guiding spirit in our creative lives. ❖

David Muench

I climbed to the first ledge above Havasu Falls to capture ambient morning light on an overcast day. I used a wide angle lens to show both drainages and the incredible drop of water on the pool.